PUSHING THE LIMITS

PUSHING THE LIMITS

Success Against The Odds

Mark Eccleston
with
Andrew Quirke

Psychology News Press
London

First published in 2007
by Psychology News Press
9a Artillery Passage
London E1 7LN

psychologynews@hotmail.com

Set in Palatino
by Keyboard Services, Luton
keyboardserv@aol.com

Printed in by Biddles, Kings Lynn, Norfolk

Distributed by Melia Publishing Services
Godalming
Telephone 01483 869839
melia@melia.co.uk

ISBN 978 0 90763 308 0

Mark Eccleston captained Great Britain at wheelchair rugby, switched to tennis and became the first British player to be ranked No. 1 in the world.

This is his first book.

Contents

Mark's Dedication

I would like to dedicate this book to Pat, Jimmy, Michael and Gary. I have – no doubt – caused them many a sleepless night as well as a load of grief over the years, but without their support and love I would never have made it to where I am today.

It is no coincidence that both my brothers have also been successful. That is simply down to the way our parents brought us up. They should be extremely proud of what they have done for us. We are certainly proud of them.

I would also like to thank Lucy for her love and support.

Huge thanks go to Andrew for listening to me rabbit on for the past two years and bringing what was first a joke in the pub with Jimmy into reality. If nothing else, it's been a laugh, mate. Thanks also to Mike Gill for getting the ball rolling.

We have included material from family and friends to give a rounded picture. So I would also like to thank everyone who contributed to this book. I asked you to take part because of the roles you have all played in my life. If I have missed anyone out, then I apologise: it wasn't intentional.

Special thanks go to Brian Worrall for being the one who gave me the kick up the arse I needed and so richly deserved. You gave me the belief and were the best coach I ever had.

To those of you out there who don't like me, it is because you don't know me – and because I don't want you to.

If I have upset anyone in this book then you need to look yourself in the mirror and ask yourself why.

He who laughs last...

I have left some swearing in the book as I feel it is relevant to that particular moment. If this offends I apologise.

I may also offend the politically correct brigade with some of the language I use in this book. The truth is I don't care. I don't care what people call me but, as strange as it may seem, I am not too keen on being called 'disabled'. Disabled implies that you can't do anything. If you disable a computer, it doesn't work. But I don't spend twenty-four hours a day in my pyjamas. Okay, I'm in a wheelchair but my serious opinion on my situation is that I am injured. I have a spinal cord injury and I am a tetraplegic. It's an injury I've had a long time and one that isn't going to get any better in a hurry, but it's an injury nonetheless. If you injure your knee, you have a knee injury. Having a spinal cord injury is not the end of your life, as you are about to discover.

Mark Eccleston

Andrew's Dedication

I would like to dedicate my work on this book with all my love forever to Emily and our wonderful baby son, Oliver. To borrow a line from Morrissey – 'Now my heart is full and I just can't explain so I won't even try to'.

I would also like to thank Mark Eccleston for giving me the opportunity to work on the book and put onto paper a truly inspiring story. My thanks as well to our agent Sonia Land for all her help, our publisher, David Cohen, Mike Gill for putting me forward, Kevin Gill for his library scouring, Carley Gee for her expert advice, Sarah and Mike at *The Bird I'th Hand* and Mum for believing!

Special thanks go to Mark's mum, his dad and his brothers.

Thanks also for giving their time and recollections to; Chris Johnson, Brian Worrall, Rob Tarr, Ian Moffatt, Jason Harnett, Adam Langley, Carl Moffatt, Jimmy Crooks, James Pankhurst, Phil Leighton, Anthony Cotterill, Jamie Burdekin, Lorna McCarthy, Dr Clive Glass, Stuart Dunne, Mark Heesome, Jim O'Reilly, Matt Lancaster, Rick Draney and Steve Smith.

They reckon you can judge a man by his friends. If so Mark Eccy is most definitely a legend as you're all top men.

I would also like to thank Sir Cliff Richard for his quote about Mark.

Andrew Quirke

Preface

I have lived in St Helens all of my life, and yet up until December 2004, I had never even heard of the name Mark Eccleston.

The man should have been a household name with all his achievements, so for me not to have heard of him in my home town is particularly shocking.

A Paralympic hero who should have been in the national press, let alone local papers, but whose achievements went unrecognised.

Meeting Mark for the first time, I quickly realised he had an incredible story to tell and that he was going to tell it in a hugely entertaining way.

Anyone who knows Mark and has encountered him in his sporting career knows just how amazing his achievements are.

It's been an honour to work with Mark and my sincere wish is that this book goes some way, not only in making more people aware of his talent, determination and drive, but also in giving wheelchair sport the recognition it deserves.

His sporting record speaks for itself, but Mark's story is much more than the sum of his outstanding achievements.

Andrew Quirke

Chapter 1

A Matter of time...

I was born on the 2nd of December, 1969. I grew up in the Clock Face area of St Helens in Merseyside. Clock Face was one of the old mining villages like Sutton Manor, Lea Green and Bold. I lived at the bottom end of Clock Face. The Clock Face area of St Helens actually came under the Widnes boundary at the time, so officially I'm a Widnesian. After I was born, the boundaries changed, but as far as I'm concerned I'm a St Helens lad. I lived there until 2004 when I finally moved out of my mum and dad's, much to the amusement of some of my mates! My mum was a dinner lady at St Teresa's school; my dad was a mechanical engineer at the Pilkingtons Glass factory in St Helens.

It's the same with any kind of area like Clock Face; some people call it close-knit, and others would use the word 'incestuous'. Everyone knew what everyone else was doing. If you wanted to know what was going on, you could spend an hour in the pub and you'd be up to speed. If you were ever in trouble, plenty of people would help you out. It was a tight-knit community. I was born in the house that my mum and dad live in to this day. When you have lived in an area for so long, part of you is glad to escape, and part of you always feels a very close association with it. It was a good place to be brought up. There were plenty of places to knock about, play rugby and get into trouble.

I used to go to St Teresa's school where the headmistress was a nun called Sister Mary. She taught my mum, my brothers and then me. I was only there a couple of years and then St Mark's School opened on Leach Lane and I went there.

St Mark's was where I started playing rugby league. There was a teacher there who was mad keen on rugby called Tony Brown. There was only a football team at the school when he arrived so he started a seven-a-side rugby team. He entered us into a tournament in Crank – yes, there is a local village called Crank – and we won the third place plate. I scored two tries in the Plate Final. Tony is now the official in charge of the video referees in the Super League.

I also messed about a bit though, like the time when I found out that if you put plastic two pence pieces from the science lab into the sweet machine it worked. I used to get tons of sweets like this and sell them on for a penny. I got caught in the end and I got in trouble big time.

They said it was theft. I said it was using my initiative!

SCRAPPING SCOUSERS

We went on a school holiday to the Isle of Man when I was about nine. On the ferry over we were all scrapping with a school from Liverpool that was also on board. Two days later on the Isle of Man itself, we saw them again and the battle recommenced.

There was a lad who I used to knock around with called Des Callaghan. I went away on holiday to North Wales with him and his gran and granddad a couple of times. We went river fishing every day and it was brilliant. There was a rope swing that went out over this fast flowing river, and I would swing out on it and dive in. An early indication of the daft things I would later get up to.

I look back at some of the stuff I did as a kid, and it would horrify me if I had kids and they did the same things.

When we were eleven, Des and I got a train from St Helens Junction and ended up in Sheffield. I only got back at nine at night. If I had a kid that age now and they took themselves off to Sheffield alone, I would go ballistic.

I did the typical stupid things you do growing up. If anyone was going to climb a tree, jump out of it or do a somersault into a haystack, then it would be me.

Inevitably, I got in a bit of trouble here and there. There used to be a bridge in Clock Face; a mate and me stood on it once, dropped our pants and pulled moonies to the school buses. We didn't know but the number 23 bus came past with some old lady on it. She was that horrified at what she saw, she went to the school and reported it. The school launched an investigation into who were the two boys showing their arses on Clock bridge and it didn't take long for the trail to lead to me. I got collared for it. They sent me home with a letter to my parents, and I was grounded.

I had no fear as a kid. There would be times where other kids would say 'I'm not doing that' and I would do it, no problem. I went to Coniston with St Cuthbert's and I would walk along the top of waterfalls. I would sit on top of them and quite happily dive in, even though there was about a 20-foot drop to the rock pools.

Let me fill you in on more of my stupid stuff. A couple of my mates had pellet guns and we used to go over the fields shooting rats. This one day a lad shot at me in the leg so I grabbed the gun off him and told him he had until I counted to 10, then I was going to shoot him. He started to run and I counted to 2, then shot him right up the arse!

He was rolling around on the floor screaming at me, 'You said you was going to give me till 10.'

'I can't count,' I replied.

We nearly nicked a train once. At Sutton Manor Colliery, the trains used to park at the siding by the tip. Des was a train buff and knew his stuff.

Someone left a door open on this train and we got on and Des then looks around to try and start it. We'd have been off with it if he could have got it going, but we got chased off.

Forget robbing cars, this was major league, 11 years old and trying to hotwire a Class 47 diesel train.

We also used to go to Spike Island in Widnes and swim in

the lock that joins the canal to the River Mersey; it is about fifty foot deep. Someone dared me to jump in it starkers, so I did. They then chucked my clothes in which was a bit of a nightmare considering it was the middle of summer and the place was packed.

We'd also go rock climbing at Pecks Hill without any equipment; we were like monkeys. Proper climbers, with all their gear on, would look at us in horror as we scampered past them up the rock face.

We'd go to the apple orchard and rifle as many apples as we could. Getting the apples was like a military operation; there would be shouts of 'cover my back' as we darted between trees.

We'd steal potatoes from fields and then sell them. We'd get chased all the time. We'd throw stuff at the lads who sniffed glue under the motorway bridge. I don't know what else was in the glue, but those lads would chase us for hours. We'd throw rose buds at people's windows. That wasn't too bad, but it went too far when someone threw a brick.

If someone did the same to me now, I'd cut their nuts off. I did well at school despite all this larking and my growing fascination with girls. In my fifth year, just before exams, we had one particular teacher, Mr Bradbury. We were always clashing, and he was always rollicking me. There was this one day when we were all silent doing a mock exam. Sat at the table next to me was a girl I used to go out with on and off all the way through secondary school.

She had the biggest breasts in the year. They were magnificent! I had this flexible ruler and I bent it back and let it go on her baps. She let out the loudest scream you have ever heard; then she went nuts and started to attack me. The teacher called me out to the front of the class. 'Eccleston you clown, get out here,' he said.

He couldn't resist giving me a lecture in front of the whole class. The subject being I was a loser as well as a clown and, therefore, I had no chance of passing the O level. I thought it was a bit out of order so I asked him if he wanted to have a bet on it.

4

I suggested that he put his money where his mouth gabbed. We agreed that if I passed the exam he would give me a fiver, and if I got an A or a B he would give me a tenner. He said, 'Easy money Eccleston, you've got no chance.'

We shook on it in front of the whole class.

I took up boxing for a while at St Helens Star. I was heading for my first amateur fight when I had to make the choice between boxing and rugby. Rugby won. This was probably the earliest indication that I preferred a team sport to an individual one. The boxing school was disappointed I left. Years later I saw one of the trainers; Tonka (who fought professionally) said I would have made it as a boxer. He still calls me 'champ' when he sees me now. My mum was glad I gave up boxing though: I think she was scared of me ruining my good looks!

I ended up falling out with Des Callaghan as we went to separate secondary schools and started hanging out with different lads, and I heard he'd been slagging me off.

I saw him one day and asked him if he'd been slagging me off. He said he had. We started fighting, well, he threw a lot of punches; I remember it was a Thursday and 'Top of the Pops' was on. As he was throwing punch after punch, I asked someone the time and they said '5 to 7'. 'Top of the Pops' came on at 7 so I threw one punch. He reeled away with blood gushing from his nose and it was all over. I just walked off. I hated fighting but could handle myself if I needed to.

I also had a paper round after school that paid three quid a week. I used to run round and use it as part of my rugby training. One of the places I delivered to was a truck haulage place that had three dogs, two huge Great Danes, and a little Jack Russell. These three crazy bastards used to attack me every single day. I'm sure they used to sit down and plot how they would get me because the two Great Danes would always corner me – and then the Jack Russell would come in for the kill and latch itself to my leg and wouldn't let go.

Another place I delivered to on the paper round was a kennel and cattery at the end of a lane where young lovers would park up in their cars and do their thing.

5

In winter, when it was dark while I was delivering, I would creep up the side of the fields behind the bushes and sling eggs at the cars as they were 'going at it'.

Got chased loads of times doing that.

RUGBY LAD

After St Marks', I went to St Cuthbert's High School (Cuthies), and it was full on rugby there, the only problem being that they moved me from position to position. I played wing, then full back, and I was fed up because I wanted to be in the middle where the fur was flying. It was at Cuthies that I started to become really good friends with Ian Moffatt, known as Moff.

Ian Moffatt

I got to know Mark Eccleston (Eccy) at senior school. We both played rugby league so we instantly connected. I don't mind admitting we were the best players on the team. We used to go watching St Helens RLFC together too and, in the year of the great Australian star Mal Meninga, we were ball boys at Knowsley Road.

Our French teacher at St Cuthbert's, Jim O Reilly, set up a rugby team outside of school and it was based at St Helens rugby club – nicknamed Saints. Between us we got the Crusaders side started. We got some players from other schools down and ended up with a good team. We played there for three years. Eccy made me go out on ridiculous 8 mile road runs every week to get fit. He was nuts but always very determined and focused.

It was a battle between Eccy and me for the player of the year. Crusaders used to train at Saints on a Thursday night and that was the night they had Saints' disco, so after training we would head there. We had some good laughs and pulled loads of women!

Eccy was a legend when it came to the girls.

He would always go for the athletic girls at school and had some success despite his penchant for wearing Val Doonican jumpers.

We used to do lads' things together like 'budding' where you would get rose buds, throw them at windows and get chased.

We used to play rugby in the streets and enjoy a couple of beers during this time as well. We also drank home brew or cans of Royal Dutch, every Saturday when my parents went out.

But Moff and I were serious about rugby.

Jim O'Reilly, the French teacher at Cuthies, started up the St Helens Crusaders amateur Rugby League team. We got some decent results, but the top teams at the time were Leigh Rangers, Woolston (who were basically the Warrington town team) and Blackbrook, which was St Helens town team in all but name.

I went down training with Moff down to Blackbrook a couple of times but it was very cliquey. They wouldn't speak or pass the ball to us, so that's when Crusaders started.

Steve Ganson, the Super League referee, used to play for us, though he was a far better ref than he was a player. He was terrible on the field and had a Billy the Fish mullet hair cut.

I remember a French school that came over one time. Mr 'Bonky' Barrow was coach of the school team a year above me and asked me to play for them against the French. It was a big deal if you played for the year above so I was thrilled when he asked me.

However, it seemed like everyone in my year was there watching and during the game he shouted, in front of everyone, 'I believe you're a hard tackler, Eccleston, so prove it son.'

So I thought I better had – or I really would look like an idiot.

I waited till the biggest French player took the ball up and I laid him out fair and square. I then turned to the coach and asked, 'Will that do?' I was cocky then as well.

We didn't have a brilliant team at Cuthies but got to the semi-final of the schools town cup in 1984. If we had won we'd have played the final at Saints' home ground, Knowsley Road. We lost.

I really wanted to make it as a rugby player; we would play all the time and I used to get Moff to come on mad training runs all round Widnes, which would take us hours.

We used to go watch my brother play at Widnes Tigers under 19's; they were a great side and that would psyche us up. Great also meant they were a tough outfit and partial to the odd fight or two. We loved it. Tony Karalius, brother of the Saints legend Vince, coached them and they won everything.

Moff and me would get on the home brew at his house, and get the girls round when his mum and dad were out, as they were every Saturday night.

We trained at the Saints pitch on Tuesday and Thursday. Thursday was great as afterwards there was a weekly disco. The girls would be stood at the window watching us train and, of course, we would all start showing off. There was a presentation night coming up and the players agreed that we had to bring a girl to it. At this disco was a gorgeous girl we all fancied by the name of Tracy. We were all stood round saying, 'I can't ask her', as young lads do.

I marched over and asked if she would come with me; she said 'yes'. The other lads were astounded. The story spread like wildfire and at school the next day I was 'the man'.

I would be asked, 'Have you really got Tracy to go the presentation with you?'

My answer was like Finchy out of American Pie, 'Yes, yes I have.'

I was king dick. The only person I forgot to tell was the girl I was sort of seeing at the time!

That ended our relationship.

At the presentation night, my date ended up copping off with Moff! He still goes on about that to this day, the slimy sod. But I respond by telling him that technically he had my sloppy seconds. I did all the hard work and he went in for the kill. I was gutted. But I did end up going out with her mate, who was quite fit, but also slightly bonkers.

One day, Moff and me had both girls back at his and were in Moff's bedroom. The next thing Ted, Moff's dad, walked in and caught us literally with our pants down.

What do you say? 'Hiya Ted, are you OK?'

Needless to say, Ted was not impressed and sent me packing. If you're at all sports minded in St Helens, then talk soon turns to rugby league. Both my brothers played rugby league to a good standard with the pair of them representing the town. My oldest brother, Michael, was more into athletics and was a good runner. My other brother, Gary, played rugby for Lancashire and was selected for Great Britain trials; he also played a few games for Saints reserve team.

So, it was a natural thing for me to go into rugby league. I was a pretty good player. In fact, we were due to have the St Helens Crusaders Player of the Year awards and it was going to come down to between me and Moff for player of the year.

The presentation night was set for the same day as the FA Cup Final between Liverpool and Everton in 1986. I asked Jim O'Reilly whether I was going to get a trophy. He said he couldn't tell me. I said if I wasn't getting an award, I wouldn't be going as I had a ticket for Wembley.

He said, 'You'd better turn up.'

I thought, 'Yes, I've got it.'

The last game of the season I played well but Moff had a stormer. He was a great player, fast, with a good pair of hands, and while you could tell his dummy was coming, he'd still do you with it. Moff won Player of the Year and I was runner up. The chairman at Saints was John Clegg and he presented us with our awards. When I collected my award, John Clegg said, 'Stay with us lad and we'll see you right.'

I was later told by someone involved in St Helens RLFC that if I was to stay on and play for the Colts, there was a chance they would sign me on. I don't know if this was true but it was what I was told.

We had a few coaches at Crusaders who had good standing in the professional game such as Eric Chisnall, John Butler and Dave Mackay. I flitted between hooker and loose forward until we got a lad who could only play hooker so I stayed in the back row. I was a good ball handler and could play anywhere in the pack. Mackay was sure that I would make it as a professional; in fact, he once told me he thought I would eventually play for Great Britain. Whether he said this to build my confidence I don't know, but what I do know is all I ever wanted to do was make it as a professional.

That's the biggest thing that eats away at me. I'll never know how far I could have gone in rugby league.

When I left St Cuthbert's I got offered a couple of engineering apprenticeships and eventually decided to take one at Simon Vicars, a big engineering firm based in Newton Le Willows.

It was August 1986.

THE WORST HAPPENS

I had time to kill before starting my apprenticeship. Nowadays, you go to college and university, but, back then, you went into an apprenticeship. I finished my 'O' level exams in June. I wouldn't start at Simon Vicars till the end of August.

And where better to kill time in the summer than in a haystack?

Every summer we used to mess about at the back of our house where there was a big farmer's field. There was a big tree there and we used to put a swing up on it.

It was a Sunday. As I was coming out of the door my mum asked me where I was going.

I told her 'the swing' and she replied, 'Someone's gonna get hurt over there one day.'

I just said, 'Yeah, yeah, whatever', went out the door and climbed over the railings. My mate was fixing his motorbike and told me he would meet me at the swing.

We were jumping out of the tree into this big haystack we had put together. We were just bored really. I had done it every summer a million times before. There was a steep embankment leading to the field and I ran down it and attempted to do a somersault into the haystack, but I didn't time it right. I landed straight on the back of my head.

There was no dramatic cracking sound, like you hear on TV when someone breaks his neck – just a strange, painful sensation like an elastic band snapping. I knew straight away, and said, 'I've done my fucking neck in.'

10

I lay on the haystack with my chin tucked into my chest and my voice started to go really high pitched.

I was saying to my mates, 'I've done my neck, I've done my neck', but because I was always messing about they didn't think I was being serious. I lay there for what seemed like an eternity telling them I wasn't joking. I couldn't move. I was totally paralysed and my whole body was tingling with pins and needles, and if that wasn't bad enough, I was now struggling to breathe.

My mates kept telling me to get up, but I couldn't.

The way I got them to believe that I couldn't feel anything or move was to tell them to start pulling the hairs on my legs. One of my mates did just that. He was pinching me, but no matter how hard he pinched, I never reacted. Finally they realised I wasn't joking.

One of the lads ran off to get my mum but he said that when he ran across the field, he kept looking back; he was expecting it to be a joke with me leaping up any second.

No chance.

My head was tucked into my chest, my voice was suddenly high pitched and I was now gasping for air.

I told them again I couldn't breathe and that they were going to have to move me. They did so. Not one of us knew that if you have a spinal injury, moving you is the last thing anyone should do.

I always remember my mate Jimmy, a few years later, after a few beers, brought it up and told me he felt guilty about it. I told him not to because, if he hadn't moved me, I would probably have died, as I was hardly able to breathe. I was a bit upset that he had kept it to himself for so long; if he had said something straight away I would have cleared it up for him. The fact I was moved may, or may not, have worsened my injury. That's something we'll never know. But what I do know is that if I had not been moved, I would probably be dead.

SHAVED BUT SAVED

The ambulance came down the farmer's track, as the swing was

11

an awkward place to reach by road. The feeling of pins and needles was getting more intense and I was beginning to realise that I had done something really serious. But I felt no pain. It was bizarre: breaking my neck never actually hurt.

But I knew I had done something bad. They put me in the back of the ambulance. As we left my estate, I told the ambulance driver to turn the sirens on to give the neighbours something to talk about. I also remember getting to Whiston Hospital. They had to cut my clothes off. I was going mad at them saying they couldn't cut my T-shirt off. As they cut my top off, they were pulling straw out as well.

The next day I was transferred to Southport Spinal Injuries Unit at 5 m.p.h. under police escort. We had to go that slow due to the nature of my injury. The next thing I recall was somebody shaving my hair. I had long, thick hair and, because I was a vain little sod, it used to take me ages to comb it.

I went mad when they started to shave my hair. I asked them what they thought they were doing; they told me they had to shave it. I was furious, but there wasn't anything I could do as I couldn't move a muscle.

After shaving my hair, they injected me, cut me and then drilled into my head. I wasn't happy with the injection, as I am petrified of needles. They put on traction but there was no improvement in the alignment of the dislocated vertebrae at C6, C7 level. So it was decided to manipulate and reduce the dislocation.

Mr Soni, the consultant, carried out the operation and reduction was achieved without difficulty. To maintain the reduction my neck was extended and traction of 5 pounds applied. It was determined that my diagnosis was C8/T1 Tetraplegic (traumatic) with 50% forward dislocation of C6 over C7 (bifacetal dislocation). In non medical words, I was up the creek without a paddle; in fact, I didn't even have a boat.

I had dislocated two vertebrae in my neck and severed my spinal cord.

I was drifting in and out of consciousness. I could hear talking, I was so blasé about it, I wasn't screaming or anything,

I was more of the attitude 'Oh God, what are you lot doing now?'

To be honest, I was still seeing my arse over them shaving my hair and giving me the needle. They must have given me something knock-out-strong at this point, as I don't remember a thing after that.

THE SMELL OF HOSPITAL

When I came round the first thing I noticed was this horrible smell. When you're on traction you have this wishbone thing clamped to your head. It is fixed onto a rope and pulley, they put weight on it to pull the bones in your neck apart, and then take the weight off gradually to bring them back together. That was seven weeks on my back staring at the ceiling. Just imagine seven weeks when you can't move and the view never changes. The boredom was total. I actually made an extremely feeble attempt at killing myself.

I pulled the blankets over my head one night, thinking that would be enough to suffocate me and that I wouldn't wake up. I was extremely annoyed to be awoken in the morning by a nurse.

But my mood did soon change when she said she was going to feed me my breakfast – and then give me a bed bath to which I replied, 'I'm not hungry love, so crack on with the wash!'

My mates were gutted when I would point out that this particular nurse (who they all fancied) that very morning had my family jewels right in the palm of her hands. That bed bath was more than adequate compensation for my ridiculously pathetic attempt at killing myself.

So that I could watch the TV, mirrors were arranged to let me see the end of the bed. Initially, I couldn't move at all. I knew something was wrong and I kept asking the nurses why couldn't I move my legs?

Jimmy Crooks – *Mark's best mate*

I was with him when he had his accident, I actually moved him because he was suffocating. I was one of the first of his mates to see him in hospital; it was pretty bleak seeing my mate like that. He was still strapped to the bed. He was very bitter for a while, but that was to be expected.

The spinal unit was near the marine lake in Southport, and I used to get the mirrors fixed in such a way that I could watch the boats sailing on it. I would watch the lake all day. All I could see was the sails going past but it was exciting, a lot better than staring at the ceiling.

I had just started getting a bit of movement back in my arms and I was asking what was wrong with me all the time, but the nurses kept putting me off. Eventually I found out why. My consultant was away on holiday; they were waiting for him to come back so he could tell me what I had done to myself.

The accident had happened on a Sunday. When I came round I thought it was Sunday evening and I kept saying, 'I've got to go training at Saints on Thursday, when am I getting up?' Those weeks I spent in intensive care, that whole experience, I could write a book about that alone. So many life-changing things, bizarre things, happened.

One good thing was that I got my 'O' level exam results while in intensive care. It was quite the occasion really with loads of people stood round my bed wanting to know how I had done. I passed seven of them and was thrilled, as I'd been worried that I had messed up. Fair play to Mr Bradbury too, I got a B in history and he sent a cheque for ten pounds to the hospital.

I saved the money till I could get down to the pub.

Oh yes, I got drunk on that ten pounds. Cheers Bradders!

I learnt a lot of stuff that had nothing to do with school, as you do when you are 16 and paralysed. There were four of us in that small room. There was a girl next to me who was only 17. She was from Scotland and had come down to work in Blackpool. Some lad had given her a lift in his car, but he had been drinking and ended up hitting a lamp post. In the bed opposite her was a bloke called Stuart who had been injured playing football. He was paralysed from the neck down. Then there was a policewoman who had fallen off a horse.

Later an old bloke called Walter joined us. I will never forget him or his wife. He was clearly oblivious to where he was or what was wrong with him. His wife was this tiny frail old lady and she would come in every single day, sit next to his bed and talk and talk and talk to him. She was a lovely woman and it was heart breaking to watch her do this every day. She used to tell him everything was going to be OK but she had no idea of the enormity of his situation. It was pitiful to watch at times; he would never reply because he didn't even know she was there.

Because you spend so much time with these people in such a small space and you're all going through the same agony, you get to know each other quite well. There are no secrets. I got to know Stuart's two kids who would come over and feed me.

It was a surreal experience. You're on the bed, they come in every morning, wash you, roll you, feed you, put cologne in your hair to stop it going scabby. You get into a routine. Smells were important actually. Even now I can go somewhere, catch a whiff of something and it will make me think instantly of my time in hospital or intensive care.

While I was in intensive care, about seven St Helens Rugby League players came to see me. My uncle also managed to get me a huge get well card signed by Liverpool FC and all the top players like Dalglish and Souness. Sadly, it got robbed. I kept it with my O-Level certificates and they both disappeared.

My consultant finally turned up, a top man by the name of Mr Krishnan. He asked me if I knew what I had done and I replied that I knew I had damaged some bones in my neck and that was why I couldn't move.

He then asked if I had any questions.

All I was concerned about was my rugby and I asked him if I could go training on Thursday, as I was sick of lying around and the season was starting soon.

Mr Krishnan told me, very matter of factly, that I would never play rugby again.

Talk about a kicking a bloke when he is down.

I went mad.

I asked him why I couldn't play rugby again. He said it was because I had damaged my spinal cord and that it was very unlikely that I would walk again.

My mum and dad came in after Mr Krishnan had spoken to me. I was crying.

I said I had just been told I was never going to walk again. My parents both cried. It's the first time I'd ever seen my dad upset. That was hard, that sort of thing eats away at you. He was telling me not to worry, that everything would be okay but I knew that wasn't the case. I don't remember a great deal after that.

The nurses told me afterwards that they sat talking with me over the next day or two, but I have no memory of it. They say I was talking about girlfriends, rugby and school but I just don't recall any of it.

Right by the hospital there was a church. My mum had never been inside it but she decided to go in to pray for me. All of a sudden she heard someone call out her name. She turned round to see Sister Mary. The last thing she expected was to bump into the nun who used to be her teacher back in St Helens!

Sister Mary came to see me quite regularly at the hospital after that. I still get a letter off her at Christmas; she is in her 90s now and lives in Birmingham.

THE TRUTH ABOUT MY INJURY

I came round and began to ask how long I would be lying in intensive care. I was told six weeks – and after that they would start getting me up gradually. One of the physios told me that my injury was a level higher – i.e. worse – than it actually was. I was neurologically a traumatic C8/T1, and she was saying I was a C5/C6, which is even more severe and basically means you aren't going to be doing as much for yourself. I was left wondering whether I'd ever be able to dress myself, go the toilet without help, work or have a girlfriend. It was only after talking to a nurse one day that I realised my true level of injury. I understood then that I would be able to do all these things. She told me that they had treated people with the same level of injury in the past and they managed to live on their own.

In a perverse kind of way, the physio did me a favour as I went from thinking I would have no independence in the future to realising that wasn't the case at all.

They always tell you the worst-case scenario in hospital because if you get any more function back, it's a bonus. It was a kind of buzz realising that I was going to be able to do some things for myself.

They moved me out to the next ward along although I was still on my back in traction. To make things even worse, when I was in intensive care I'd been having trouble sleeping. The nurses gave me some medication and I ended up tripping off on it. Hello hallucinations! I thought there were snakes crawling over me. Other times I thought I was on a conveyor belt and they were building a car round me, so I was grabbing hold of the traction and I actually tried to pull it off.

Moff was the first person to come and see me after my family had done. They weren't going to let him in at first but he explained he had come from Aintree – and in his dinner hour – and that he was my mate.

Ian Moffatt

I was the first of Eccy's mates to see him after his accident. Straight from leaving school, I went on a hotel management course at The Park Hotel in Aintree. I got a phone call off my mum telling me that Eccy had broken his neck. Eccy was my mate and I just couldn't believe it. We used to train together, play rugby together and go on long mad runs together.

The chef of the hotel dropped me off at Southport.

I got out of the car and walked into the hospital. Eccy's mum and dad were heartbroken. I was crying and they said they didn't want Mark to see me while I was in such a state.

I walked in and Eccy broke down in tears. He said, 'Throw me out of the window, I'm a spaz, I don't want to be here.' It was awful seeing my best mate like that. He was in intensive care with clamps on his shaven head. It was shocking.

It broke my heart to see how upset he was. He had lost everything as a result of doing something that thousands of kids do.

When I visited him in hospital, he would lie in his bed exercising by grasping his hands. He couldn't even look out of the window. He couldn't move his head when he was in traction. He didn't want anyone treating him differently and he got a bit of an attitude about it. I could understand where he was coming from. This was a very fit lad we are talking about who had just lost everything in a split second and that's just how he dealt with it.

I didn't know anything about spinal injuries. You don't until it affects you. I just thought that the hospital would be able to help him recover fully. That's where Eccy's strength came in; he told me one day to quit telling him that he was going to be all right.

He told me he knew he was not going to be OK and to just have a look round the ward, as it was full of cripples.

He told me they were not going to walk again, so why should he?

Moff was a hard lad but when I got upset he had to walk out because he just couldn't take it. Later he told me he went outside and had to be comforted by a nurse as he was crying his eyes out.

When they came in to tell me they were going to take my traction off, I was made up. Then I got thinking that it had been on for seven weeks and with the hair and scabs it was going to hurt like hell when it was removed. There was a lad in the ward who kept going on about how painful the moment of removal was.

Mr Soni came in to the room. I'll always remember that a Prince concert had been on telly the night before. Mr Soni asked me if I had watched it, and I told him I had.

He then asked me if the concert was any good, and as he did so, undid the bolt. The traction sprang apart, ripping itself away from my head.

I was about to answer his question but, instead, proceeded to scream loudly.

Now that DID hurt!

My head was throbbing like mad. I could feel the blood trickling down the side of my face.

'All done now,' Mr Soni said very casually and walked off.

A nurse had to come and patch me up.

LOSING WEIGHT

A couple of the girls who used to go the Saints disco visited me too. Fair play to Tracy, she came nearly every week.

The nurses started raising me up bit by bit, day by day. When they put me up I nearly fainted because I had been on my back for so long. I had also lost a lot of weight. I think I was about eleven stone when I went into hospital. Three months later I had dwindled down to around eight stone.

The girlfriend of one of the lads I was in hospital with went over to Australia and this was at the time I was getting into Australian Rugby League. I would watch the latest videos from over there. Brett Kenny was one of my favourite players and I asked her to get me a Parramatta jersey, as he played for them. She brought me one back. It fitted me then but when I look at it now, it probably wouldn't fit my seven-year-old nephew. That's how much weight I had lost.

From when I can remember, I have always been fascinated by Australia. My auntie lived out there and maybe that sparked off my interest. When I got my apprenticeship, I told my mum and dad that, as soon as I qualified, I would be going over there.

Obviously, that was not going to happen now.

Chapter 2

Starting from Scratch

There was so much for me to deal with – and I was only 16. Dealing with such an injury is not easier now but medical technology has progressed. Back then it was pretty brutal – from having your head shaved, being injected, then drilled, to having something sprung from your head. The worst thing I'd ever done before was when I broke my nose playing rugby.

I broke my nose twice actually; my mum told me to get it straightened but I told her it was a momento of my exploits on the field!

The first time I broke it was when we were playing Bulldog at school on the carpeted sports hall. We had a teacher who was straight with you. He used to give you the old 'bacon slicer' with his cane if you did anything wrong. Even today, if I saw him, I would call him 'Sir' – he just inspired that sort of respect. We used Bulldog as rugby training and with us tackling on carpet, you would always come out with friction burns. I was picked to go in the middle on my own, with forty odd lads running at me trying to get past. One lad had been annoying me all day so I thought I'd go for him. I got my technique wrong and his knee got me flush on my nose.

My God the pain was incredible!

My nose burst. This teacher came running over saying, 'Eccy, Eccy.'

I said, 'Fucking hell, sir, that hurt.'

He said, 'Less of the language and get off my carpet. If you stain it you are on detention.'

There was blood pumping out of my nose, I couldn't see as my eyes were watering so much and I was in total agony. But all he was concerned about was the well-being of his shag pile!!

I went to hospital and he later checked on me. I said I was okay.

Sarcastically, I enquired after the purity of the carpet, only to be told that it wasn't stained. I had, therefore, escaped detention.

There was a lot to deal with in the aftermath of my accident, like someone shoving a finger up your jacksy to empty your bowels, or shoving catheters down your penis so you could have a wee.

When you're 16, things like that are very hard to handle. You've also got to deal with seeing your family upset. I would later learn the doctors had told my parents that they were a bit concerned about a blood clot I had. My mum stayed in the room at the hospital. One night as she was giving me sweets, I started choking; then I coughed up this massive blood clot. It was like something in a cartoon. The clot seemed to fly across the room in slow motion, waving at me!

To see your family having to deal with all this is pretty hard. Mentally, it makes or breaks you. You either give up, whinge about it and have people look after you for the rest of your life – or you meet it head on. Fortunately, my personality and upbringing instilled the attitude that I was never going to give in.

I have seen a lot of people have their spirits broken by such a severe injury. Believe me it's not a pretty sight.

I have seen grown men cry and give up. There was one man who had the same level injury as me, but he had given up. He kept his arms in the same position for so long that eventually he couldn't straighten them. When the physio came to work on him, he would scream. I'd shout at him, telling him not to be such a wimp. I was just a kid and he was an adult, but he had abandoned all hope and I just couldn't listen to any more of his whinging and screaming.

His wife and kids would visit; he would tell them that he didn't want them to come and see him. That must have been awful for them.

When I started getting up, it was horrible. I was feeling unwell all the time and vomiting. I went back into the intensive care ward to see Stuart whose injuries were so bad he could only communicate by tutting. Not long after that, he died.

Stuart's death affected me. I had spent six weeks in intensive care with him and his wife and kids would visit every day but I have never seen his kids since. It's very difficult to go through an experience as traumatic as being in intensive care with someone, only for them to die soon after. I still think about how they were then, Paul at six, and Lisa who was about eleven. I wonder where they are now and what they are doing.

I spent seven months in the spinal injuries unit. Strange as it may seem, I look back at some of that period fondly. I was the youngest one on the ward, and I used to get all the attention. I was looked on as the baby so nurses spent more time with me. They used to mother me a little and believe me I milked it, big time!

Some experiences were extremely unpleasant though, and I had to grow up very, very quickly.

I saw things I didn't want to see and I heard things I didn't want to hear.

It was horrible.

Once I started getting up though, that's when reality hit me right between the eyes, and I really found out what it was all about. It's like you are a baby and are starting from scratch, learning everything all over again, how to wash, get dressed, feed yourself, go to the toilet, almost how to breathe.

Even though I am a positive person, I wouldn't wish what happened to me on anyone, not even my worst enemy.

If you're not mentally strong enough and you don't have strong support around you that kind of trauma will see you off, especially if you are as young as I was.

I hadn't been up in bed long and someone who worked down the gym asked me how things were going. This person asked me if, when I was pushing down the ward and I saw some of the nurses, did I get aroused?

I could not believe they asked me this.

23

I thought 'right you are having it'.

I replied, 'Too right I do. Have you seen such a body? I wouldn't mind getting into her.'

They just sat there gob smacked, you could tell they were not expecting this response, especially not from a 16-year-old kid.

I thought it was such a bizarre thing to ask me so I went on for half an hour about all the nurses and what I would like to do with them. They didn't know what the hell had hit them. It was funny. In the end I was ushered out of the gym even though I hadn't quite finished. They never asked me that question again.

I had my accident in the August. I was in bed the whole of September and the majority of October. When I finally got up, it was dark and unpleasant so I wasn't able to go out much.

BACK TO THE WORLD

Before you're discharged from hospital the staff take you back into the big wide world, only this time you are paralysed and it's oh so different.

I remember the first time I went out. The spinal unit was about a hundred yards away from the Lord Street shopping area of Southport. One of the occupational therapists took me out. I hadn't had my hair cut for months and it had grown pretty long, so I asked if she would take me to the barber's. Not long before I had my accident, the BBC's school drama, 'Grange Hill', screened the first episode to feature someone in a wheelchair. This was a very big deal at the time. I'd always liked the show, and now it seemed to speak directly to, and about, me. They had this storyline about two kids in wheelchairs going to the school. It's not as bad now but back then people used to stare at anyone in a wheelchair. I did it myself before my accident and think 'I wouldn't like to be like that'.

Anyway, this occupational therapist took me out, and as we pushed towards Lord Street, a gang of kids walked towards us. I heard one of them say, 'There's that lad out of Grange Hill.'

I got upset and asked to be taken back to the ward. I didn't get my hair cut that day.

I had been worried about going out in public and the very first time I did, *that* happened. Anything like that hurt me more than any of the physical pain; it really affected me. I went to pieces and I hid in my bed. It stayed like that when they started allowing me to go home for weekends because I just didn't want to leave the ward.

I did stuff to make sure I didn't go home and the easiest one was pretending I was ill. The first time I went home I was very nervous. OK, you had people coming to visit you in hospital, your family obviously, your mates and so on.

But what you have to remember is the last time I was at home I was on my feet, active, able, a rugby playing jack-the-lad. Now I was going home in a wheelchair. Also they didn't have the modern design of wheelchair that's available today; they were big, clunky contraptions back then – like tanks – and you couldn't push them on your own. There would be loads of people who hadn't been to the hospital seeing me for the first time. I was dreading it.

I asked my dad to pick me up when it was dark because I didn't want anyone to see me getting out of the car. When I got in the house it seemed like the whole street was there. I know they meant well, but I hated it and just felt like I wanted to die.

Then my mates came and took me to the Clock Face Hotel pub. People were nice but you could tell some felt awkward talking to me. They'd say 'hello' then go off quickly. I just remember thinking that when I got into the pub, I was going to get very drunk because I didn't want to be there. I wanted to blank it all out. And yet I was used to it.

When I was in hospital, part of the therapy was to take you to the pub. The thinking was: get you out of the ward and into the big wide world. Going to the pub aged 17 with a load of nurses was exciting. My mates and some of the nurses took me out into Southport for my birthday; it was the first time I had ever been into a nightclub. It was a very good night as I got very drunk and pulled a stunner. The pub was packed.

However, back in the Clock Face when I went in, it was like Moses with the Red Sea, everybody parted for me. What's more, they started clapping. 'Who the hell are they applauding,' I thought. I found it very upsetting.

I just wanted to go back to hospital. I had been told I was to spend the rest of my life in a wheelchair and they were clapping me? I was really uncomfortable with that, thinking, 'Haven't I got to achieve something first before I start getting applause?'

When I went home that first time, it was too much for me and I got wasted on Southern Comfort. My hangover was so awful that I have never been able to even look at a bottle of the stuff since.

After that, I made excuses so I wouldn't have to go home. I just couldn't stand being there. I'd feel like a circus freak, especially as there was no one else who was in a wheelchair. I'd be sat in a pub and I could see people having a look over at me and I felt very uncomfortable. You'd get the looks and the stares and then, when you made eye contact, the awkward smile.

I harmed myself in hospital in an attempt to stop going home. I put a mark on my backside once and I scratched my penis. When you have a spinal cord injury it affects your bladder. Back then they would put condoms on you with a hole in it, all attached to a leg bag. These condoms used to mark my penis so I used to rip them off to leave more of a mark, so I wouldn't have to go home. I did that two or three times until the nurses realised what I was doing.

And visitors came when I was home. We didn't have a big house back then, so three or four people in our front room was claustrophobic. I hated that and I hated going to Clock Face Hotel pub.

THE PORSCHE OF WHEELCHAIRS

It helped to get rid of my tank of a wheelchair and replace it with a snazzy red sports model. It was the most expensive wheelchair available at the time, costing about £2,000. The Porsche of wheelchairs made life easier for me. If I was going to travel in a wheelchair, then it had to be the best one available.

Mum (Pat) *recalls*

Mark's got some good mates and they've all stuck together. When he was in the hospital he didn't want the NHS wheelchair so three friends of mine; Jean Moffatt, Joyce Richards and Dot Welding organised a concert for Mark at Sutton Labour Club. This helped raise the money to get him a sporty wheelchair.

Being a kid, I wanted to show off my new wheels. My mates would come to the hospital asking what the chair was like. The people of Clock Face were fantastic in that they did a lot of fund raising for me, like Mum said. A couple of lads also ran marathons for me. It was incredible and I will be eternally grateful to them. This new wheelchair gave my confidence a massive boost.

But hospital had become comfortable, too comfortable.

I wanted to stay 'inside' because I wasn't unusual there, the nurses didn't look at me any differently, the doctors didn't either, and the people visiting didn't, because it was a spinal injuries unit – and being in a wheelchair was the norm.

Then something critical happened. I kept on being told about this lad who had the same injury as me, and yet could do all kinds of stuff. Alvin came in on a Wednesday to play table tennis. I saw him and could not believe how low the backrest was on his chair.

I eventually got to meet and talk to him properly. And he was an inspiration. Let's start with how to behave in bed.

One of the real pains of being paralysed was that, initially, it would take an hour to get into bed.

To prevent you getting sores in bed the nurses would put pillows under your feet, under your back and between your legs. I asked Alvin how many pillows he had in his bed and between his legs.

He just laughed and told me the only thing he ever had between his legs was a woman.

'Brilliant!!' I thought, 'I'm having some of that.'

He told me everything he did, and showed me how he got in and out of his car. I asked him if he could do a back wheel balance, and he pulled a perfect wheelie right there in front of me. I was gob-smacked.

He had the same level injury as me, yet he was shagging, driving, even clubbing. The magic penny dropped. I wasn't going to have to be a sack of potatoes for the rest of my life.

I still see him every now and then. He probably doesn't know this, but he was very instrumental in me being driven to be as independent as possible. He had been told the usual stuff of how the injury would limit him, yet he defied all the expectations. He broke all the rules in the spinal injury handbook.

It's progressed now and people who have the same injury look at me and see what can be done. I just thought that if he could do it, then so could I. The new wheelchair and meeting Alvin happened at the same time. That's when I stopped doing stupid things to myself and felt more comfortable going home.

I still didn't like it though.

In March 1987, I was discharged from hospital and I moved into a residential home in Weld Road, Birkdale until an extension was built at my parent's house. I spent seven months at Birkdale but I'd go home for days. My mates would also come over and stay and we would go out into Southport and party.

I saw a lot of things in my months in hospital that could have broken me. I had become institutionalised and, like the hospital had been, Birkdale was also getting too comfortable. Again people in the same predicament surrounded me. Once I was out of that comfort zone, I found it very hard to adjust – so much so that I became quite arrogant, bitter and aggressive.

I upset a lot of people during this time, especially my family, and for that I am really sorry.

There were still things I couldn't do for myself. I couldn't get my pants on, no matter how hard I tried. I couldn't go on the toilet on my own, which I found difficult to handle. Here I was 17 years of age and I needed someone to help me have a dump. It was awful.

At Birkdale there were less staff, so it took them longer to get round to helping you. It was a blessing for me though because I'm quite impatient, I thought to myself, 'I'm not waiting around for them to come and help me', and subsequently, I learnt to do everything for myself.

When I left there, I was independent. The sense of achievement I felt when I eventually went to the toilet for a dump without any help was incredible. And that was not the only skill I mastered. I also got fit there.

I used to go out pushing in my wheelchair every morning. In the end, I would go into town on my own on a Saturday night. In seven months I had gone from not wanting to go outside at all to going out on my own, aged 17, and getting pissed in town!

I arrived at the conclusion that I was stuck in a wheelchair and as much as I hated it, I couldn't do a damn thing about it. You have the choice of staying in and being unhappy or going out and having a good time. I opted for the latter.

TABLE TENNIS

Dad (Jimmy) *recalls*

When he was in intensive care I went for a walk round the hospital and watched a couple of lads in wheelchairs play table tennis. I went back to Mark and told him about this, he said 'how can you play table tennis in a wheelchair?'

After Dad told me that I went down and watched them play. Soon after I joined the hospital table tennis team which was, of course, a wheelchair team. We competed in a league, in which all the other teams were able-bodied or AB. At first, I expected the AB's to take it easy on a little bloke in a wheelchair. Like hell they did!

The Able Bods played to win, which was exactly what I needed. If they didn't care about beating up on a bloke in a wheelchair, then that was fine by me. I wanted them to smack it by me as hard as they could because, believe me, if I got the chance, I was going to smack it at them back.

When I went to rehab the physios wanted me to do weights. I would get the weights over and done with as quickly as possible so I could play table tennis because I loved it.

Every year, the National Wheelchair Games are held at Stoke Mandeville near Aylesbury. It's the home of wheelchair sports. While I was in Birkdale, one of the lads from the sports club at the hospital took me down there. I won silver at table tennis; the following year I won gold and was the National Champion. They were good weeks because they were so eye opening. All the wheelchair sports were on show and you could see what was available to you. The games also included a good drinking session.

I saw lads like Stuart Dunne from Cyclone wheelchairs, who is a good mate of mine now. He had the same level of injury as me. I watched what he could do and learnt a lot. There were also women hitting on me left, right and centre – which was a bonus. The second year when I won gold, I got introduced to wheelchair rugby. Although I enjoyed table tennis, it was too static for my taste. I wanted movement and action, and so table tennis wasn't a long-term option for me.

When I eventually got back to St Helens I had a hard time with a couple of mates. A few of them just didn't know how to handle the situation. One even crossed the road when he saw me so he didn't have to speak to me. I spoke to him eventually and he said he felt guilty because he just didn't know what to say. When something like my accident happens you soon find out who your true mates are. When I started going out properly, we would go to a lot of places that had steps going into them.

I used to feel bad about my mates having to lift me in and out of these places.

I once asked my mate Jimmy if he got pissed off having to lift me up and down steps. He said it would piss him off even more if I didn't come out.

Little things like that mean a hell of a lot to me.

Even though society back then didn't really know how to take people in wheelchairs, it was a bit easier in Southport; people were more used to seeing wheelchair users because of the Spinal Unit.

With certain people I had to go to them. They had never experienced anything like dealing with someone in a wheelchair before and didn't know how to react. I struggled more with that than I did with any of the physical challenges. Lifting weights and getting fit are controllable. If you want to push up a hill, you can will yourself up it. You are in control of that. But people's attitudes you can't control and, although I'm not a control freak, I do sometimes struggle with what is uncontrollable.

MY FIRST GIRLFRIEND AFTER THE ACCIDENT

From the moment I was first told I would never walk again I was worried about my chances of finding a girlfriend.

In early 1988 I began my first relationship since the accident and the way I handled what happened did nothing to ease my initial concerns.

After I got home me and my mates would go to the disco at Thatto Heath Labour Club every Friday night because it was full of women.

This girl kept looking over at us and she was gorgeous. Regardless of what my mates would say I would not have it that she was looking at me.

Anyway, this girl that walks over and says 'Hi are you Eccy?'

Aye Aye here we go!!

It turned out she worked with a couple of girls who I knew.

We began seeing each other and everything was going okay, although I did find it strange that she would never let me in her house. However I eventually realised why when her dad starts telling this joke about how cannibals looked upon people in wheelchairs as meals on wheels!

Everywhere we went though, lads would be looking over because she was so good looking. Initially this was great as it was a bit of an ego boost.

On the other hand, it was always in the back of my mind that she would eventually leave me for someone not in a wheelchair and when lads would chat her up right in front of me, this would do nothing for my ever-increasing insecurities.

They assumed she was my carer or nurse and this happened a lot.

She was also the kind of person who enjoyed a bit of attention and what could get her more attention than going into a pub with a kid in a wheelchair.

She had a birthday party and it was that night we had our first real fight, up until this point we never really argued that much.

After her birthday we would argue quite a bit and she was pretty feisty to say the least. Once she threw a coat at me and the zip caught me flush in the eye. She was helping me down three steps once and decided to let go on the last one. This girl would argue that black was white.

We went to Manchester one night and were on our way home when all of a sudden she started screaming about pain in her stomach. I drove to the hospital and then a doctor comes out and tells me that she had just had an ectopic pregnancy.

Now, due to the fact I had not yet ejaculated since my accident, I was 100% certain that she wasn't pregnant, certainly not by me anyway.

I told the doctor this but he assured me that this indeed was the case.

During our relationship I had convinced myself that she would eventually go off with someone else, so hearing this made me even more paranoid.

When she came out about an hour later she said that it was a kidney problem, but by this time it was 3 a.m and I just wanted to go home.

Subsequently she began having appointments at the hospital for what I thought was a kidney infection.

A couple of days later, she phoned me and asked me to go round her house because she wanted to talk to me. She said the hospital had told her that she might not be able to have kids. She was upset and said that she loved me and that she thought I would dump her because of it.

I told her I wouldn't dump her but all this came as a bit of a shock for an 18-year-old kid with a broken neck just out of hospital.

Anyway, the relationship went on until one night we had a big argument about Arthur Scargill and the Libyans! (Scargill was leader of the National Union of Miners and he had some very odd political alliances.)

I stormed off after this and after about two weeks she called to say I was dumped. So off I went round to the house, gutted, to collect some of my things.

When I got there she came walking out with another lad and, naturally, I was a little inquisitive as to his identity.

I started thinking back to that night in the hospital. Right there and then I convinced myself the doctor had been right, she had been pregnant and, as it could not have been mine, she had been going off behind my back with this lad who now stood before me.

My theory was compounded 12 months later when I drove past St Helens Hospital and saw her at the bus stop with a rather big belly, and this after she told me she might not be able to have kids.

The ironic thing was she spotted me looking at her from the car and SHE gave me the finger!

I have since realised that my paranoia and insecurities made me wrongly arrive at the conclusion she had been messing around and that it was purely because I couldn't walk. But I was 18, just out of hospital and, as far as I was concerned, if anything negative happened to me at this time, especially where women where concerned, then it was because of the wheelchair, end of story.

She may or may not have been going off behind my back, the doctor may or may not have been right, that's irrelevant, but going into a relationship paranoid that I would eventually get dumped because of my wheelchair meant that it wouldn't have lasted anyway.

It never occurred to me that maybe I was dumped because she didn't fancy me anymore or the relationship had just fizzled out. As far as I was concerned, and nobody could convince me otherwise, she had dumped me and done the dirty on me because I was a poor little cripple, and because of my immaturity on this issue, I turned into a very bitter young man.

I was tapping off with women all the time and I would arrange to meet them and not turn up.

I would arrange for them to meet me at a certain place and I would drive past just to see how long they would wait for before they left. In my eyes it was a revenge thing – and revenge is not the noblest of things.

Even IF she did do the dirty on me, which I now know she never, I shouldn't have reacted the way I did. But I was just 18, I had convinced myself I wouldn't get a girlfriend because I was in a wheelchair and it was my way of being defensive.

But that's still no excuse for the way I behaved. So if you were one of those girls who waited ages in the freezing cold for me and I never showed, I apologise.

I have matured since then and although at the age of 18 and fresh out of hospital I thought all women would dump me because I was in a chair, I soon realised that plenty wouldn't, and the ones who would just weren't worth bothering with anyway.

MY BIT FOR SCIENCE – ECCY THE GUINEA PIG

Another thing I did around this time was go and see Mr Krishnan and ask him if I could have an RGO walking brace. The RGO (reciprocating gait orthosis) is a set of callipers that enable you to stand up and walk, or wobble, around. I just thought 'I'm not going to walk again am I? I'll soon show you'. I had seen a lad using one at the spinal unit and I wanted to try it out.

Mr Krishnan told me that he was very reluctant to let me try it, as I didn't have enough balance and my injury was too severe. Nobody at my level of spinal cord injury had ever done this. However he recognised my determination and said I should be allowed to try. I was sent to Hope Hospital in Salford for an assessment and tests.

They agreed to let me on the program. The first time they stood me up I blacked out. Learning to use the brace was a very long process. They make you stand up each day, for a little longer each time. Eventually, I would walk round the hospital and to the car; eventually I was allowed to take it home and used it nearly every day.

I was asked to be the best man at my mate's wedding and I was determined that I was going to learn to stand and walk in time for the big day. On all the wedding photos you can see me standing up.

Ste Smith, *the groom, remembers*

It meant everything to me when he stood up by my side as best man for my wedding. I didn't think I'd ever see that. He's unstoppable when he puts his mind to it. That was such an achievement and it tells you what sort of person he is. There's none of this 'well I've got this far that will do' attitude with him. He sets himself a goal and he gets to that goal. I don't go out for a beer with him so much these days due to family commitments and the fact that there's no such thing as going out for 'a beer' with Mark; there's usually a few beers involved!

I have done my bit for science too. Around 1993 I did a study at Salford University with a Saudi Arabian guy called Anil and a physio. They used electrodes to stimulate the muscles in my legs. They were looking to see how much energy I was using when walking. Anil told me he went to a seminar of the world's top people in this area at Glasgow and told them what he was doing with a tetraplegic. They wouldn't believe it until he put the video on. He said as far as he was aware I was the first tetraplegic in the world to do this and no one thought it was possible.

Walking was hard work though. The benefits of being able to stand up are obvious, but I am not too sure about the benefits of walking for a tetraplegic. Being paralysed affects your muscles and joints and they just aren't the same. I've got osteoarthritis in my right hip and I do wonder if it is a result of walking in the brace.

It took me about four years after leaving hospital for me to pluck up the courage to go out drinking round St Helens town centre.

I was worried about seeing anyone who knew me from school. Once I got over that hurdle, however, I was fine and would go out every Friday, Saturday and Sunday. There would be girls turning up at the house too, girls who I'd gone out with at school. I was kind of going out with a girl when I had my accident (the one in history with the big baps!), but it had been on and off really. She passed word on through my mates that she was going to come and visit me at the hospital but she never turned up. I don't think she could handle it.

She eventually turned up at the house one day when I was home and we started going out again. I thought it was going well till all of a sudden she stopped it, giving me some excuse about going on a training course. Again I put it down to being in the wheelchair.

I saw her a few years later and I asked her why she stopped seeing me. I explained it had done my head in because I had been out with her at school and she had been one of my first relationships after the accident.

Fair play to her, she was upfront about it and said it was because she was 17 and was worried about the sex thing. That was something we hadn't discussed. I asked her why she hadn't asked me about it at the time; she said she was embarrassed and found it awkward.

At the age of 18, and when you are in a wheelchair, these things really bother you. People believe that if you're in a wheelchair you can't have sex or have kids. I thought that myself as no one at the hospital had spoken to me about it. It was a knock to my confidence when she dumped me as I convinced myself that it was because I was in a wheelchair. I started to wonder whether this was going to happen all the time.

Eventually, though, being in a wheelchair became an ice-breaker if anything. Girls would come over, talk to you, wanting to know what had happened. It usually took about 15 minutes before the conversation got round to sex.

A lot of the time when I was younger, girls would say, 'Oh, you're dead good looking, it's a shame.'

I would sit there thinking, 'if only you knew'.

Maybe they thought I was getting more rejections than Osama Bin Laden at a Thanksgiving bash, but that couldn't have been further from the truth.

I have always been one for challenges, and the subject of women and sex certainly was a challenge back then.

I do like challenges. But every single day for the past 20 years I have wished my accident had never happened. I have accepted life in a wheelchair and all the baggage and bullshit that comes with it, but that doesn't mean I have to like it.

In fact, I hate it. Big time.

Chapter 3

What My Friends and Family Felt

When I eventually realised the implications of what I had done I became consumed with self-pity and bitterness. I am the first to admit I became angry with the world and developed quite a chip on my shoulder. My situation also affected those around me, especially family and friends and those who cared for me. But at the time I just didn't realise how much.

Mark's Mum (Pat) and Dad (Jimmy) *recall*

Pat

Mark knew straight away there was something seriously wrong as he kept asking the nursing staff, 'Why can't I move my legs?'

After his accident, there was one day he was sat in his chair by the window and saw some kids heading in the direction of the field where it happened. He asked me where they were going. I went upstairs and looked out to see they were going to the swing over the field. He went out and went to town on them because he knew what could happen.

Jimmy

Mark used to go to a boxing club as a kid he and did all right at it too; he would have been good at any sport. He was due to start work the week after his accident.

Pat

I like most sports but I'm not a boxing fan and wouldn't have wanted to see Mark get hurt. I watched him play rugby league too although I used to shout too much!

When he first came home after his accident, my instinct was to mother him but he never wanted any help. If he wanted help he would ask for it, but he gets annoyed at people who offer him uninvited help.

Gary, *Mark's brother*

Before the accident, he was just a typical teenager. I think he would have been a very good rugby league player. He was still at school when I was working but I was hearing good reports about him. After the accident, he became more focused, he had tunnel vision, and if he wanted something he was going to get it. He had a lot of hard times but there was no stopping him once he knew what he wanted.

I'm very proud of what he's overcome. I don't know if I'd have been able to do it. The way he adapted and got on with life is a credit to him. His philosophy seems to be that he has been dealt the cards he has – and he has to get on with it.

Mike, *Mark's brother*

The period immediately after the accident was obviously traumatic. From visiting Southport hospital and the half-way house during Mark's convalescence, I thought that Mark and people in a similar situation would either 'do something' or 'do nothing'. Mark clearly decided to 'do something' and he changed quite quickly. He has always been quietly confident and determined, but after the accident he became even more determined and confident in himself, almost aggressively so.

I would use the analogy of a very gifted rugby player with all the natural speed, confidence and flair in the world, but without the determination and aggression required to be 'the very best'. In my opinion Mark became 'the very best' almost overnight. With this he also grew-up very quickly.

Jim O'Reilly, *teacher at St Cuthbert's*

I remember the first time I saw him in hospital his head was in a clamp, he was looking in a mirror to look around and he was obviously very down. As time went on, you could see the improvement in him, not so much in his physical condition but in his way of mind. When he came out, he made his mind up that he was going to get involved in wheelchair sports and achieve at the highest level. I am full of admiration for the way he adapted to his condition.

Ian Moffatt

I quit rugby when Eccy had his injury; my head was all over the place. I restarted playing through a few lads who were at Thatto Heath asking me to play again. Ironically it was in the same team as his older brother, Gary. Within half a season, I was getting picked for Lancashire and Great Britain amateur Rugby League. I ended up going on tour with Great Britain. I always thought though if I was doing this, what would Eccy have done? He was a very good player and he would have made it professionally.

Ste Smith, *friend and neighbour*

I was in Spain at the time of Mark's accident. I'd gone away with a group of lads from college. When I came back, my mum told me and I was devastated. I didn't go to see him in hospital at first because I didn't know what to expect. It took me another two months to go and see him because I just couldn't do it. When I did see him I thought he had started to get his head round it. What he's told me since is that he hadn't at that point. He thought his life had come to an end and he was just putting a brave face on it. He used to play football and rugby with us in the street, then all of a sudden he's stuck in a bloody wheelchair for the rest of his life. He could have sat there and said 'right, this is me, I'm in a wheelchair and everybody else can feel sorry for me' but he's not, he's took it by the scruff of the neck. I really, truly believe because of the way he throws himself into things that he would have become a top rugby league player. If he hadn't played for

Saints, he might have, God forbid, played for Wigan. He would have been at the top of his game.

Lorna McCarthy, *physiotherapist and a friend*

The first time I met Mark was in a pub, strangely enough! It was not long after his accident and we had gone to take some of the patients for a drink. My sister, who is a nurse at the spinal unit, introduced me to Mark and we started chatting. During the course of our chat I said to him, 'On your bike', and he said, 'I wish.' I just thought, 'Oh my God, I can't believe I have said that.' I was only young myself at the time. He was quite mean really. It was understandable though as he was so young.

We've had a few alcohol sessions I have to say! We used to go into Southport, drink, push the patients back to the unit, give them back to the night staff and leave them to it! If someone asked me to remember some really good times it would be that period. We were a group of young girls, all single, no ties, who used to go out an awful lot. Some of the younger lads who were also patients would come out with us.

Mark was very much the baby of the bunch. He could charm anyone; he got attention without any problem. He was the favourite of all the nurses.

But he could be very hard work as a patient. The one thing I would say is when he got involved on the sports side of things he very quickly had the determination to get the best out of every part of rehab. He was so focused on anything that he needed to achieve. Even though I can give him a hard time for being very bitter when I first met him, quickly he became very mature.

He is one of the most determined people I have ever met and as an athlete one of the easiest patients I have ever dealt with. He has one of the strongest characters you can imagine and an amazing will to succeed. At the time of his accident, there were lots of other lads in wheelchairs who received financial payouts as the accident was someone else's fault. Mark didn't get anything like that. His family were so lovely and were there day in, day out. They were so supportive. Some people when they have been in hospital for too long start criticizing it but his family were never like that. They were filled with respect and gratitude.

What Friends and Family Thought

When I first met Mark, he could very easily have gone the other way and given in. If you'd have asked me which way I thought he would go, I wouldn't have known. He was angry with life, everybody was talking about what could have been with his rugby league career and endless might-have-beens. Mark believed, however, that there were more opportunities out there. He picked up very quickly on the potential that there was more to life than him sitting in a wheelchair and giving up.

Chapter 4

Murderball

Every year the National Wheelchair games are held at Stoke Mandeville. Dave Hickson, who was in the sports club at Southport, picked me up and took me down to them in 1988.

It was the first time I got to see wheelchair sports apart from table tennis.

Wheelchair rugby was one of the most dramatic. Its roots go back to 1977 when it was created in Manitoba, Canada, specifically for quadriplegics.

Back then wheelchair basketball was the most common team sport for wheelchair users. It required players to dribble and shoot baskets and that relegated tetraplegics athletes, who have functional impairments to both their upper and lower limbs, to supporting roles. The new sport, originally called *Murderball* due to its full-contact nature, was designed to allow tetraplegic athletes with a wide range of functional ability levels to play. The sport includes elements of wheelchair basketball, ice hockey and handball. Physical contact between wheelchairs forms a major part of the game.

Wheelchair rugby is played by two teams. Four players from each team may be on the court at one time. It is played indoors on a court of the same size as a regulation basketball court, 28 metres long by 15 metres wide. The court has a centre line and circle, and a key area measuring 8 metres wide by 1.75 metres deep at each end. The goal line is the end line of each key.

Players score by carrying the ball across the goal line. For a goal to count, two wheels of the player's wheelchair must cross the line while the player has possession of the ball.

A team is not allowed to have more than three players in their own key while they are defending their goal line. Offensive players cannot remain in the opposing team's key for more than 10 seconds and a player who has the ball must bounce or pass it within 10 seconds.

Teams have 15 seconds to advance the ball from their back court into the front court. Physical contact between wheelchairs is permitted but some aspects are deemed dangerous and forbidden such as striking another player from behind. Direct physical contact between players is also not allowed.

In some cases, a penalty goal may be awarded instead of a penalty. Common fouls include: *spinning* (striking an opponent's wheelchair behind the main wheel axle, causing it to spin horizontally or vertically), *illegal use of hands* or *reaching in* (striking an opponent with the arms or hands), and *holding* (holding or obstructing an opponent by grasping with the hands or arms, or falling onto them). Wheelchair rugby games consist of four 8-minute quarters. If the game is tied at the end of play, 3-minute overtime periods are played. Competitive wheelchair rugby games are fluid and fast-moving, with possession switching back and forth between the teams. The clock is stopped when a goal is scored, or in the event of a violation, such as the ball being played out of bounds, or a foul.

As in all wheelchair sports, players use custom-made sports wheelchairs that are specifically designed for their sport. Key design features of a wheelchair rugby chair include a front bumper, designed to help strike and hold opposing wheelchairs, and wings in front of the main wheels to make the wheelchair more difficult to stop and hold. All wheelchairs must have spoke protectors, to prevent damage to the wheels, and an anti-tip device at the back. Electric wheelchairs aren't allowed.

The wheelchair rugby ball is identical in size and shape to a volleyball. Wheelchair rugby balls are typically of a 'soft-touch' design, with a slightly textured surface to provide a better grip. The balls are normally over-inflated compared to a volleyball to provide a better bounce. Players use gloves and adhesives to assist with ball handling, and various forms of strapping to help them keep a good seating position and balance.

To be eligible to play wheelchair rugby, you must have some form of disability with a loss of function in both the upper and lower limbs. The majority of wheelchair rugby athletes have spinal cord injuries at the level of their cervical vertebrae. Other eligible players have multiple amputations, polio or neurological disorders such as cerebral palsy or some forms of muscular dystrophy.

Players are classified according to their functional level and assigned a point value ranging from 0.5 (the lowest functional level) to 3.5 (the highest).

When I eventually got classified, I was given a 3.0 rating or a 3-pointer.

The four players on court at any time for a team can't be 'worth' more than 8 points. If you played three people like me, for example, the team would be insufficiently 'disabled' as we would total 9 points. The classification process begins with an assessment of the athlete's level of muscle function. An athlete must have a neurological disability that affects at least three limbs, or a non-neurological disability that affects all four limbs. The athlete then does a series of muscle tests designed to see the strength and range of motion of his upper limbs and trunk. After the player gets his classification officials watch him play in competition to confirm the way he plays reflects what was observed during muscle testing. Usually doctors, physiotherapists or occupational therapists do the classifying.

The first international wheelchair rugby tournament was held in 1989 in Toronto, Canada, with teams from Canada, the United States and Great Britain. In 1990, wheelchair rugby first appeared at the World Wheelchair Games as an exhibition event, and in 1993, the sport was recognised as an official international sport by the International Stoke Mandeville Wheelchair Sports Federation (ISMWSF). In the same year, the International Wheelchair Rugby Federation (IWRF) was established to govern the sport.

As I had played rugby before my accident, watching a game

of wheelchair rugby at Stoke Mandeville was fascinating. I immediately realised I had found the sport that was perfect for me.

I began training with Southport.

THE SOCIAL TRIES TO HELP!!!

When I eventually went home to St Helens I had all these people coming round – social workers and the like. They irritated the hell out of me. They were telling me what I needed and what I should do. One came round who was your stereotypical social worker that you would see in *Viz* magazine. Ginger hair and beard, round glasses, patronising, know it all.

Ginger Know All asked me what my main aim was in life. I said I wanted to live on my own. He asked me how much a loaf of bread cost; I said I didn't know. He then asked me how much a pound of bacon cost and, again, I replied that I didn't know. He said, 'Well how do you expect to live on your own if you don't know these things?'

I think I told him to go forth and multiply and get out of the house. My mum rang them up next day and I never had another social worker visit me again. For me, personally, they were a waste of time.

Another big mistake I made when I went home was listening to a careers officer who told me the best thing would be for me to go to college. As wheelchair sports hadn't really taken off back then, I reluctantly agreed.

So, humbly in my wheelchair, I went to a college in Liverpool, every day for two years. It was the biggest waste of two years in my life. I did a Btec national diploma in Business and Accounts and cruised it, no problem, but it's been of no use to me since. At least I did get to meet a lot of people and being in Liverpool was fun, having a laugh with the scousers.

In the second year of the course, I started training a bit more and a bit harder at wheelchair rugby.

Then, out of the blue, I got a letter inviting me for the

Great Britain trials, which were being held in Sheffield. I didn't make the team to go to Canada, but I thought someone must have seen something in my play to even invite me to take part.

DEATH MAKES IT CLEAR

My brother and his wife had been talking about going to Australia for the Great Britain rugby league tour. I told them I couldn't really afford it and, also, I had decided I was going to finish my degree in Business & Accounts.

Then something happened that totally changed my way of thinking on a lot of things.

There was this lad that I came all the way through infants to high school with, by the name of Andrew Hevay. He was in the same class as me from day one and he was also from Clock Face. We hung around in the same group of lads and got on really well. He was a top, top lad and also a very good snooker player.

We used to enjoy going to the Labour club every night to play. I was not too bad at snooker, but no match for Andy. I don't think I ever beat him.

Andy knew how to live life to the full. He was always out partying and he would have three or four girls on the go all at the same time. One weekend, he went up to the Lake District camping with a few others from Clock Face. And, then, tragedy. He went out on Lake Coniston on a boat and drowned.

They brought his body home to his parents' house in Clock Face. I'd never seen a dead body before. I went through the front door into the living room, said 'hello' to his mum and dad and they asked me if I wanted to see him. I said I did and headed off to the kitchen, thinking he was in there. They asked me where I was going and told me I had gone past him.

He was in the living room in his coffin. I had completely missed him! Bleak as the day was, they had a laugh at me.

I went to his funeral. There were hundreds of people there. It was testimony to how well liked, and what a great lad, he was.

His death was a waste of a fantastic young life and should never have happened. He was a lad who really knew how to enjoy himself.

I didn't really want to do the degree course but felt pressured into it by people who were supposed to know what they were talking about.

But after Andy died, I decided I was no longer going to do something I did not enjoy. I quit the degree course and told my brother I was going to Australia with him. I also got more into the wheelchair rugby. Sport was the path I wanted to go down.

Ever since, I've never done anything I don't enjoy. I still think about Andy to this day.

THE FARMER'S TRACK

Over the road from where my mum and dad live there's a farmer's track. We used to go over there as kids stealing conkers and the farmer would come out and chase us off. I went to see him and asked if I could go on the track to push up and down it in my chair. A steep hill on his land went down to a stream and I wanted to climb it to get stronger.

He said it was fine and I was there every day. I would push up that hill ten or twenty times. Sometimes I would do it in a morning, go home, then come back in the afternoon and do it again. I would go pushing for miles. When Southport Spinal Unit opened their own training facilities I would train there as well.

I was now playing wheelchair rugby for Southport, and we went down to Stoke Mandeville and played in the national tournament.

Then in 1991 I made the Great Britain side for a tournament in Dallas, USA. It was an amazing feeling to be told you are going to represent your country – that was until they told me that I had to pay for it myself!

I had to fork out for the flight and hotel. Back then playing for Britain was more like playing for a club. You got picked but you had to raise your own money if you wanted to go.

To be honest, it wasn't that difficult to break into the Great Britain squad, as there weren't that many good players back then. You've still got to play well though. That's when I realised I was good at it and was going to give it my undivided attention.

The Great Britain coach was Brian Worrall, a man I didn't get on with at the time, although now I hold him in the highest regard possible.

Brian has been a major influence on my career. He had been one of the best players in the country. I used to go after him all the time and try and get the better of him, but he would show me up and I didn't like it.

America was a good laugh, exciting and a lot of things happened on that trip that determined what kind of player I would become.

I know it sounds like I am blowing my own trumpet but, towards the end of my rugby career when people were sat round discussing who the best players in the world were, my name would usually come up. I was by far and away the best player in Europe. There were a lot of great players in America and Canada but they had a much bigger population of wheelchair users to choose from.

DALLAS TRIUMPH

Dallas was the defining moment though. While I was there I realised I could become one of the world's best tetraplegic athletes.

The Number 1 player in the country at that time was another 3-point player from Birmingham and here I was, a 21-year-old who was as cocky as a rooster at dawn.

I thought I should have been playing instead of him. I shouldn't have been but it was the way I felt at the time. As a new boy, being so young, I was far too full of myself.

I didn't realise that I was not going to play that much, and was just going for the experience. I was really annoyed that I was not picked for any of the matches.

Like at all tournaments, they always had a slap up celebration dinner and the one in Dallas was at our hotel. We had one match to play – the morning after the dinner. Some of the American players and staff said they were having a party back at their hotel round the corner. I wasn't going to miss that. I went round and it was wild. Two American staff members, who picked us up at the airport, were there and they partied like animals who'd just been let out of the zoo. You didn't expect the girls who picked you up on the happy bus from the airport to be so lively! At the age of 21 I was in a foreign country with a load of girls taking their tops off.

I had quite a good night.

I left the party and rang my mum up from the girls' room. It was 4 a.m. and I was very drunk. Those were the days where I could get drunk, party till the early hours and then get up and still play well. Stamina was my middle name. I was known for it.

I got to the tournament next day and Brian told me I was starting!

I said, 'No problem.'

IN TROUBLE OVER GIRLS

We were watching the match that was on before us. One of the girls from the night before came walking past and shouted, 'Hey, Mark, great party last night. What did your mum think of you ringing at 4 a.m.?' Brian, the Great Britain coach, was sat nearby, and heard her. He looked at me and went mad! That was it. He investigated the party. When we got back to the hotel we were all told to go to our rooms and wait for Brian to ring.

Eventually I was summoned up to his room.

I couldn't have cared less. I was pissed off that I hadn't played much and I had the impression that he didn't like me anyway.

When I got there, Brian was furious and reminded me that I was there to represent my country – not to stay up till all hours partying.

He told me I hadn't played much because I wasn't good enough. He said in no uncertain terms that if I ever pulled a stunt like that again he would make sure I never got picked for Great Britain again.

I realised I had made a big mistake and apologised. That was in February 1991.

When I got back home I began to train a lot harder. I realised I had a lot of work to do if I was to break into the national team.

That conversation in the hotel room in Dallas was the almighty kick up the arse I needed to get my act together. I took over the training at Southport. I showed them all the moves we should use and both myself and the team started to improve.

In 1992, I went away with GB Wheelchair Rugby to Canada. I still didn't get much game time, but it was here where I hooked up with my mate Rob Tarr. He played rugby for East Midlands and we hit it off straight away on the field – and off. He'd been on a lot of these trips before and he knew where the best bars were. He also introduced me to my first strip club, called Filmores, in Toronto. I just could not believe what I was seeing. Nothing like that went on in St Helens.

Rob was banging out dollar after dollar getting the girls to dance for him. I was gob-smacked by it, especially as they were all stunners.

Back on court, I got a write up in the Daily Telegraph because I played in the last game on the tour and got the man of the match award.

Rob Tarr – *Great Britain wheelchair rugby teammate and roommate*

First of all, let me say that I think my contribution could move this book from the middle shelf to the top shelf.

I first met Mark at the Ludwig Guttman Sports Centre at Stoke Mandeville in the late 1980s. We were both hooked on the game Murderball, later to be known as Wheelchair Rugby.

Pushing the Limits

I played for the East Midland Marauders.

As our sport is full contact, there is no time for niceties. We spent the day bashing hell out of each other and I had the impression that Mark had a chip on his shoulder, an arrogant swagger. Later that evening all the teams descended on the bar. Everyone mixed, exchanged stories and eyed up any potential female talent.

I knew several of the Southport players and was introduced to Mark. I found that we had a lot in common and his presence on the court was a way of showing his confidence in his abilities and his will to win.

We developed a firm friendship, and became drinking buddies and sexual predators, but we still kicked the shit out of each other on court.

There have been several memorable moments both on and off the courts.

There were two major events held at Stoke Mandeville, the National games held in July and a month later the more prestigious International games.

We slept in a 24-bed dorm, got pissed every night and played Murderball every day with hangovers. A huge beer tent was erected, and a disco held every night. All the local girls would come over to watch and party with us until the early hours.

Mark and myself did our best to pull as many of the girls as humanly possible. We were in and out of the tent all night.

On one occasion a very large lady approached me and asked if I fancied taking her outside. She was a little too much for me to handle alone, but I knew just the man to help me out.

I told Mark to meet me at the showers as I had a surprise for him. I am a few years older than Mark but he was always happy to follow my lead.

When he arrived I was waiting in a cubicle with this mountain of a woman, she was a man-eater and eager for us both. Mark's eyes nearly popped out of his head when he saw her, she dragged him in and shut the door.

She sat on a plastic chair in the corner with us next to her. There was a moment of nervous expectation and, then, she calmly took off her top and bra and dropped a pair of 40 double Es into our laps.

These babies were bigger than beach balls. Mark's face hit the floor. She then insisted that we do something with them.

We looked at each other, all the time doing our best to suppress a giggle.

Having got no reaction from us, she suggested we move mouth to breast.

It was at this point Mark decided to leave ASAP. As he left, things got a bit scary and I too thought it was time to abandon ship so to speak, but by this time she had fallen off the chair and was blocking the door.

I was beginning to panic as she said her back had gone and I thought I was there for the night.

In desperation I tried lifting her, using the shower as leverage. Of course, I ended up turning the shower on and drenching us both.

We finally emerged like two drowned rats. There was Mark sat outside and laughing his head off.

MVP – MOST VALUABLE PLAYER

I became player/coach of the Southport team that entered the National Championships in June 1992. We cruised it, beating everyone. At the presentation Brian Worrall gave me the trophy and told me I was the 'MVP' (most valuable player).

It was at this point that I realised that Brian had just been trying to make me a better player. The rollocking he'd given me in Dallas had provoked exactly the positive reaction he was looking for.

That hotel room in Dallas is where I believe my journey to being the best in the world began. Brian Worrall has been definitely, without any doubt whatsoever, the biggest influence on my sporting career. He knew how to handle me and get the best out of me. A lot of other coaches I worked with just didn't have a clue.

Brian Worrall – *Great Britain wheelchair rugby coach*

I first met Mark around 1986. I was playing wheelchair rugby for Oswestry and at about the same time they were setting up a team in Southport where Mark was. He was about 17 at the time, and a little hot-headed. I'd been in the Forces and you could see Mark had a bit of that in him, maybe from his rugby past. I'd been a Paratrooper, and could see a rugby spirit in Mark. He never wanted to lose. Unfortunately at that age, I had to teach him some lessons. He got too wound up. I tried to help him not to lose focus and not to succumb to the red mist, which used to happen to Mark quite a lot in those days.

His first tour in Dallas saw him partying till 4 a.m. the night before a game. To be fair though it wasn't just him. The team blew it really. On the first day, we performed quite well and then over the next few days I could tell, something wasn't right.

I ripped strips out of them later as any coach would.

SHAMELESS OUT EAST

Two days after the 1992 nationals, I went off to Australia on the Rugby League tour with my brother and his wife.

I was terrified beforehand. It was Australia, on the other side of the world, and I had never been away from home for more than ten days previously. In the past, when I had been away with Great Britain, I'd always had a physio or someone with me who knew my medical situation. If anything serious happened, they would know what to do. Now I was away with my brother and his wife who could hardly be expected to be experts in spinal injuries medicine.

We went to a couple of meetings in Leeds to meet the organisers and other people who were going on the tour. They were really good and made sure the hotels were all accessible for me.

The flight was a bit of a nightmare. We stopped in Paris, then Amsterdam, then Abu Dhabi, then Jakarta. It took over thirty hours to get there.

Former rugby league players Len Casey, Peter Fox, Eddie Bowman and Roger Millward were on the tour with us. Indonesia was something else. I think anyone with a disability there must have been shot, as they didn't know how to deal with me at all. They didn't have an aisle chair to put me on the plane so Len Casey carried me off on his back and made sure I was okay.

Those four weeks were amazing. There you are with over a hundred people who are of the same mind as you. I had been worried beforehand about how the other people on the tour would react to me and what they would be like. I can honestly say they were all brilliant. Everyone got on with each other and there were some fantastic nights out.

I had a room of my own throughout the tour. I got up to all kinds of mischief and met some really top people. One of the best nights was watching Canterbury versus Cronulla, then going to the League Club afterwards and drinking with Australian League stars, Chris Anderson and Steve Redfearn. We went down to the Melbourne test where there were 10,000 Brits, all in the same part of the ground. The noise and atmosphere were incredible. We out-sung the Aussies big time. That was one hell of a night.

The Aussies got their revenge in the decider at Lang Park in Brisbane. They split the Brits up, put us in different parts of the ground, and the locals were hostile to say the least. They would piss in beer cans and throw them at us. Fosters it wasn't. I also had the bizarre experience of hearing a familiar voice shout 'Eccy' from the stands behind me. It wasn't the booze, but a mate of my brother's!

One day we drove from Sydney to Newcastle as Great Britain was due to play the Novocastrians. We stopped off at the Hunter Valley winery area where – it was only polite – we did some wine tasting and had a barbecue. We were each given a commemorative bottle of port. As a result, you had three coach-loads of Brits drunk as skunks by the time they got to the match. With most Australian grounds, there's no terracing behind the posts; it's just a big, grass hill.

Most of the British fans didn't see the match because they were all asleep, boozed out on this hill. They showed it on TV that night. We also went to Sydney Football Stadium to see

Souths play Gold Coast who had the famous Wally Lewis in their line up. (Life is an odd thing, Wally's son, Aaron, stars in a film called 'Voodoo Lagoon', produced by the publisher of this book!)

We spent a few days in Surfer's Paradise and had many a good night at Jupiter's Casino. You look at the photos now and it's all brilliant memories as there were so many different characters on the tour.

There were all the lads from one family from Huddersfield who were like the family off 'Shameless' – shameless and good for a laugh. They'd be saying stuff to the Indonesian air hostesses who didn't speak a word of English. To be honest, it's a good job they couldn't understand what was being said. You do not want to know what these lads had in mind for these young ladies. The lads didn't speak much English themselves and I think they had tattoos on their eyes – and probably on other parts of their anatomy.

Towards the end of the tour, I wanted to get home, as it had been a long time away. I'm so glad I packed college in and went to Oz though. A tour like that will probably never happen again.

Back home I resumed training for wheelchair rugby and I was now a regular in the Great Britain set up. I had struck up a tremendous friendship with Rob Tarr. At one Great Britain training camp Brian had told everyone there was a curfew, but he would later take Rob and me to one side and say, 'Have a drink, enjoy yourselves, just make sure you don't let me down.'

He didn't give us free rein; he just gave us that little bit more. To be frank, if you tell someone they have to be in by a certain time then you don't really trust them anyway.

Brian did the right thing by giving us some leeway. He knew we would still perform. If it was a Mickey Mouse event or a training camp we would hammer the beers and come in late, and yet we would still be the best performers next morning. If it was a big tournament though, we would tone down the partying.

Brian trusted us and we appreciated that. He had been in the

Paratroopers and so knew the value of discipline, but he also recognised that we needed to let our hair down.

There was one training camp we were in and there was a nurses' social club nearby. Brian knew Rob and me would be there on a Friday and Saturday night and let it go. There are some coaches that go by the 'it's my way or the highway' philosophy and treat everyone in the same manner. Some coaches, however, are a little smarter and realise that everyone is an individual and will respond to things differently. As a cocky little 18 year-old with a bad attitude, I started off disliking Brian but while I firmly believe I would have always been a successful sportsman, he made me even better. He was the difference between my being good, and my going all the way to the top. He was just a brilliant coach and a fantastic bloke.

Brian Worral *recalls*

I probably gave Mark a little more freedom than other players. I've always had a soft spot for Mark. I could see there was a talent there and his will to win was unquestionable. I tried to steer him on the right road. Mark's the type of guy, that if you point something out to him, he takes it on board straight away and corrects the fault. With other players, you may have to tell them three or four times. As for him getting more freedom on the partying front, I don't know if that's true!

As far as playing goes, I think we're on the same wavelength. He always understood what I was trying to get across. He was pretty easy to coach. When I explained a move, he could pick it up straight away. There were a couple of other players like Mark in that respect. Rob being one of them.

He was a joy to play with too, when I was player coach.

TOO MANY PARTIES?

It may seem like I partied a lot but I trained hard all the way through to November 1992 when they had the Great Britain trials to select the side to go to North America. Brian stepped down as coach because he wanted to play, so a new coach by the name of Chris Davis came in. Straight away, he rang me saying that I was his captain and he wanted to build a team around me. I couldn't believe it, as I wasn't even in the first team at this point. He told me that I was the best player we had. I was delighted.

Nationals in the summer of 1992 had swung it for me. I had trained so hard and I had sat watching tape after tape of Michael Jordan. I would then go on court and practice all these trick passes and moves. I was spinning the ball, experimenting with moves, subtle ones, weird ones, even daft ones and also still pushing up and down hills.

By this time no one could touch me.

I worked so hard and I was cocky as well. I would do something during a game and then tell the person I'd done it to what I'd just done. However I only did it to the ones that whinged. A lot of people didn't like me because of that. In my opinion the ones that whinge about it are the ones that can't do it, or aren't prepared to put in the effort required in order to be able to do it.

People used to see the end result – me doing a flash move – but that was the tip of the iceberg. They didn't see all the hard work that went into making it look so easy.

They'd see me throw a ball twenty yards, put some spin on it, and shoot it straight onto a teammate's knee. I would do all these fakes, look one way and pass the other. It took hours and hours of practice. I would watch a lot of basketball because wheelchair rugby is similar to it in many ways. I would look at players' moves and study how I could use them in my game.

As a result of the 1992 nationals, I was made captain, and former coach Brian was also picked. The starting line up was myself, Rob, Brian and Keith Jones from Cardiff. We were something of a 'dream team'. Keith was one of the best 2 pointers in the world, Brian was one of the best 2.5 pointers and Rob was the best one point player in the world – even the Americans would admit to that.

Normally, the Americans don't give you any credit. Even in

2004 when I was in Athens, Joe Soares, a lad I used to play with in Tampa, was there coaching Canada and I met up with him. He still wouldn't give me any credit, saying I was 'an okay' 3 pointer at best.

Typical American.

When I played, Joe was probably the best player in the world, but I reckon I gave him a harder time than he gave me credit for. He was the one who gave me the most problems and I never once finished a match thinking I'd got the better of him.

He always knew how to do me over and he was the only one who could. (He was one of the stars of *Murderball*.)

In early 1993, this good line up we had went to Tampa for the 'Top End Invitational'. All the club teams in America and Canada came, but we went over as a national side. Their club teams used to be a lot better than some of the national teams. No one really knew who I was. They had seen me tagging along with the Great Britain side in Dallas but that was about it. I'd only got on the court when a game was won or lost in that tournament. No one knew what I was now capable of.

Our first game in Tampa was against Boston, one of the tournament favourites. I think we were 12 points up at half time. At the start no one was watching, but the crowd grew until it was quite sizeable as word spread that the Brits were beating Boston.

I completely ran the show in that match. I remember vividly that I had read the programme before the game and had picked out Boston's star man so that I could take him out on the court.

We ended up winning by about 20 points. I came off after the game, pushing along, and heard this voice say, 'Hey, number 33.' I looked round and saw this guy in a wheelchair with a big head and a little body, really out of proportion; he had massive glasses on too. It was Joe Soares and he said, 'Good job.'

I hate Americanisms like that; the other one they say is 'way to go big guy'.

I just looked at him and carried on going. The next couple of games we battered our opponents, and we ended up playing

Joe's Tampa team in the semi-finals. The best team in the world, they had not lost a game for ages. They were simply awesome.

WHEELCHAIR WISECRACKS

I made a huge mistake in the bar the night before the big game.

I wound Joe up. I was saying, 'I'm going to put a load of aftershave on, Joe, so when I go past you, you can smell me.'

He just sat there saying, 'Yeah, yeah, carry on.' I didn't shut up. Brian and Rob were joining in as well. Part of it was having a laugh and part of it was trying it on. We really thought we could beat Tampa – even though they were the great invincibles. Needless to say, we got absolutely thrashed. At the end of the game Joe just came to me and said, 'You should always let sleeping dogs lie.'

I had just been taught an almighty lesson. I had been cocky, arrogant and I had showed this player, who was a lot better than I was, very little respect. I got exactly what I deserved, my arse kicked, and I never did it again.

You've got to go through experiences like that to learn.

We ended up coming third in the tournament though, which was a massive, massive achievement.

Tampa was also the place where I was introduced to 'Mons Venus', the best strip joint on planet earth. It was amazing. Wherever we went Rob, as entertainments manager, would find the location of the nearest bar, nightclub and strip joint. Our coach, Chris Davis, used to tell us that we could enjoy ourselves as long as we stayed out of trouble, which we did because he was usually there with us!

The most amazing thing about 'Mons Venus' was that they had a disabled toilet in there! My local pub back in St Helens had two steps at the front so I would have to phone up before I went round, yet here I was in a strip joint the other side of the world and it was access all areas.

It was here one night that Rob had a stripper do a private dance for him. She was sat across his lap rubbing herself up and down his leg. This caused his leg to spasm, which, in turn, caused his hand to spasm. Unfortunately for the stripper, Rob had his hand on her breast. The more she moved, the more his leg went into spasm. The more his leg went into spasm, the tighter his hand held on to her. He was clamped onto her breast unable to let go. I was watching this in stitches laughing as the stripper tried to escape his clutches while, at the same time, she was screaming the place down.

From Tampa, we went up to Toronto. Again, Tampa beat us in the semi final. It was a bit closer this time but they were years ahead of everyone. Tampa had the most money and could sign the best players. For example, Joe was from Boston and they paid him to move down to Tampa.

Tampa's money came from a successful wheelchair manufacturer who sponsored them generously. They also had a bloke called Gouldie, who was the best 2-point player in the world, and an aggressive little chap by the name of Dan.

Again, we got bronze. This was huge really because no Great Britain team had ever gone over there and picked up medals: but we had won two bronzes in as many tournaments. What made it even more special was that in those days we had to find the money to fund some of the trip ourselves.

We had to pay to play for our country.

In Toronto I shared a room with Rob. You would also have people who would travel with you, nurses, physios and helpers. There was one nurse who came with us and Rob had his eye on her.

We went out one night and it was absolutely freezing, an Arctic minus 27 degrees. When you got outside, you literally couldn't speak. A few of us, including the young lady that Rob had in his sights, went to a bar. There was nothing going on with her and me but she was sat on my knee. Rob turned up and had obviously had a beer or two. He came straight over to me and punched me right in the face, accusing me of stealing his bird!

The next morning, we were in reception waiting to go out and Rob came down, looking like a little puppy with its tail between its legs. He kept saying he was sorry and I just laughed my head off.

Rob Tarr, *entertainment supremo*

I took Mark to his first strip club when in Canada. Wherever we went, as entertainments manager, my first priority was to find out where the seediest places were. However, the one that sticks in my mind is a very famous one in Tampa called Mons Venus. Tampa is the adult capital of America. Mons Venus went beyond table dancing, the girls were in your lap. One night at about 3 a.m. on our way back to the hotel Mark and I discovered we had about twenty bucks between us. As it was the end of the night, and the place wasn't busy, we managed to argue the price down and got a couple of girls. We went round the back and sat on the leather seat. We each had a girl in our lap and there was a mirror so we could see the other one. I was winking at Mark. The girl was playing around with me, and my leg started going into spasm. It's become a legendary tale over the years. That was how rugby went back in those days.

These sorts of escapades were a common thing on our trips away. I enjoyed playing practical jokes on Mark and really got him to such a state of paranoia that I only had to smile at him and he would say, 'All right, what have you done, you bastard?'

After a 15 hour trip to Tampa, Mark was busting for a dump. I gave him 15 minutes to get to his room and drop his trousers, then phoned the room with an American accent and told him we had problems with his passport; he rushed down to the lobby with his trousers literally round his ankles and suitcase packed. He found me waiting for him, pissing myself with laughter.

Over our time together he has suffered tinned peaches in his shoes, mouldy bananas hidden in his car and been fitted up with lots and lots of very dodgy women.

US VERSUS AMERICA

I came back from Tampa and Toronto in February 1993. The International Wheelchair Games were held in Stoke Mandeville that July. I was captain of Great Britain and we got through to the semis to play Canada. It was between them and the Americans as to who was best in the world. Yet we hammered Canada. I targeted their main player, and just kept on his back all through the game. It's like any sport; you figure out someone's weakness and go for it.

The final was between us and America, Joe and his lot again. We had one starting four. Me, Keith, Brian and Rob. Then you had the rest of the squad. To be honest though, if you took one of us four off and put one of the rest on, you weakened the team considerably. America, however, had three sets of four players who were all equally as good. That was the difference between us. We played them and stuck with them. They only got five points in front of us and that's how it stayed. They had beaten us, but it's the nearest anyone had come to America in a long, long time. I was gutted, though, because we had come so close.

The guest of honour at the championships was the snooker player, Steve Davis. I remember thinking that I had just slogged my balls off, got close to beating America and they made me wait in line to be introduced to a snooker player! He came over to shake my hand and I asked him what it was like to meet a star like me.

Brian was in stitches.

When the presentations ended we headed straight for the bar.

Later that evening Terry Vinyard approached me. He was the American coach – and also the coach of Tampa. He told me that he thought I had played well in the final and I told him that I thought I had nearly got them. In typical American fashion he claimed that they always had it under control.

You will never get any credit off them.

Terry asked me what my plans for the future were. I said that I was going to carry on and one day beat them. The conversation got round to whether I had ever thought about playing in America and he asked me if I liked the idea. I hadn't really thought about it up until this point, but he told me that the idea appealed to him and that he was interested in bringing me over to play for Tampa.

He said they had two teams, the Tampa Generals and Suncoast Storm. The Generals were the main team and the Storm was the second team and he wanted to get two teams to the national finals. This would be a feat never before achieved in the American league.

To qualify for nationals in America a team had to finish in the top two of their regional group. The same club can't send two teams into the same regional group but they can buy a spot in another region.

I told Terry I was interested. That was in August. I didn't hear anything from him until November when my Mum answered the phone and told me there was an American on the line for me. It was Terry.

He wanted me to be the main man in the Storm team. Twelve teams went to Nationals and Storm were ranked 17th in the USA. Tampa, of course, was the best team in the USA. I asked him how much it would cost me and he said to leave the financial side of things to him.

Terry told me he had spoken to the team and the sponsors and they all wanted me to go over and play for the Storm. They would pay for my flights and put me up for free. All I had to do was bring my beer money.

They wanted me to be there by the 7th of January ready to play in their tournament on the 10th. I trained solidly all over Christmas and New Year. Then on January 6th 1994, I headed off to Tampa.

Chapter 5

Welcome to Tampa

The arrangement was for me to stay with Dave Gould (Gouldie) in Tampa. When I got there, however, I was informed that there was a change of plan and I would be staying with another player, Mark Hickey. I'd never met him before whereas I knew Gouldie so I was a bit concerned about it.

Mark was waiting for me in his big truck. We started chatting and I quickly discovered that he had a higher pitched voice than Minnie Mouse. I remember thinking that somewhere down the line this bloke had taken an almighty kick in the crown jewels. We got to his place late in the evening.

Mark had a lodger staying there who drove a Corvette. Lodger wouldn't let us anywhere near his car, never mind in it, in case we scratched it. He went OTT over the gorgeous motor; I think it was the only car I know that was cleaned with a toothbrush. He had a nice girlfriend though who had the rather sociable habit of walking round the house naked. There was also a swimming pool, which the girlfriend went skinny-dipping in, and the pool was conveniently situated just outside my bedroom window.

Tremendous!

My problem was that Mark worked during the day so I was stuck in the house on my own a lot. I just used to watch telly all day, wait for him to come home and then go to training. It was a bit boring really, except for when the lodger's girlfriend came round for a swim.

My first training session showed it wasn't all sweetness and light. I had been told that the team had discussed me coming over and were okay with it. However when I turned up for that first session I immediately got the impression that a few of them didn't want me there. One was a lad called Steve Luzby who used to train with the Olympic high diving team before his accident. The other was Art Brewer who used to be a bouncer in Blackpool of all places!

The third was Dan, a big lad. Every time Tampa played you would notice him as the hardest player in the game. He could be nasty.

Today in most wheelchair sports you have a tip bar at the back to prevent you from falling out backwards. Back then, nobody in Europe used them, but they did in America and Canada.

I went into this first training session without a tip bar. The very first time I got the ball, Dan hit my wheel from behind and I went crashing out of the back of my wheelchair and battered my elbow on the floor: it hurt.

I thought I've been here a day and I'm going home with a broken arm!

Dan just sat there sneering at me. All his teammates were going 'yeah, Dan' and giving him high fives. I thought the situation is this – I am here a long time and if I let him get away with that, they'll all think they can walk all over me for the next three months.

However, if I get up and give him some, he may hit me, but he won't pull a stunt like that again. I got up in my chair and screamed at him that if he ever pulled a stunt like that again, I'd rip his head off and piss down his throat.

I stayed there putting on the angriest face that I could. I was expecting him to hit me. But he just pulled back, said he was sorry, asked if I was OK and patted me on the shoulder. From that point on, he was fine with me.

I feel that if I had let that situation slide, I would have had a hard time for the rest of my spell there. He could have hit me, I could have hit him back and that would have created an uncomfortable situation for a long time. I had to front up to him. By doing so he realised that he couldn't get away with that kind of thing with me, as did the other players in the team.

Most people found Dan hard to get on with but I thought he was fine. Every team Tampa played there would be one player that Dan would have a go at. He would have full-on brawls. Two blokes in wheelchairs having a fight is funny to watch, let me tell you.

The incident in that first training session probably showed my new team mates that I was serious about playing for the Storm and that I hadn't come over for a holiday. I had come to better myself and gain in experience. I also never played without a tip bar again!

That was my 'Welcome to Tampa'.

TRAINING IN TAMPA

I was never that far away from tension in Tampa. Our training centre was slap bang in the middle of one of the roughest 'projects' in the area. You had all us in wheelchairs training and gangs of black lads would turn up with ghetto blasters to watch. I think they enjoyed it. It was something different for them. In the end, I used to go over and have a chat with them as I am into R & B and Soul and they were fascinated about my coming from near Liverpool. By the time I left I'd taught all these kids loads of Scouse phrases.

I had been in Tampa three days when we played the first tournament.

First up was New York. No one gave us a chance but we battered them.

It was another one of those situations where, when every point went in, another person would come over and watch as the upset occurred. There's nothing like the underdog winning in sport. But the Americans were slagging both Tampa and myself off because they felt I had been brought in as a ringer for that one tournament. But that just wasn't the case.

We came third and, ironically, the Storm played Tampa in the semi final. Tampa were always going to win that game.

After that first session, I never had a problem with any of my teammates. But there was one issue.

I told Terry after a month that staying at Mark Hickey's wasn't really working out; he was a really nice lad but we were different people socially. I would want to go out for a beer and Mark would be sat quietly in the corner. He also worked during the day and, although we got on, we weren't really each other's cup of tea.

Terry told me I could stay at Gouldie's for the next two months. Gouldie lived an hour outside Tampa. He had been in the Navy and had been playing baseball for them when, in one game, he slid to go into base and broke his neck. He now got a big pension from the Navy. His house was massive and had a lake at the bottom of the garden with alligators and snakes in it.

The first couple of nights threw me a bit as I could hear alligator calls from the lake echo throughout the house. Once the sun went down, you could hear all the croaking. After a couple of nights though, you didn't notice it.

Gouldie had a garage in which he built a gym and it was tremendous. He also had a massive adult video collection and a staggering amount of highly educational literature.

Just to be crystal, by 'educational', I don't mean philosophy or business studies.

Gouldie didn't work so we could do stuff during the day as well. We went to Orlando and Busch Gardens and down the beach. He used to keep score for a local softball team so every Wednesday night we would go there. The team was sponsored by a bar so after the game we would head there. Gouldie didn't drink much, but bloody hell, I did. It was all free beer with food laid on and it was a riot. They were brilliant nights. He also loved the aforementioned 'Mons Venus' strip joint and he would always drag me kicking and screaming (in protest) there on the way home after training on Saturdays.

I never paid for anything while I was in Tampa. I was really well looked after. In the three months I was there I probably spent no more than £200 to £300 and that was on clothes and presents.

Gouldie liked a joke. He told me that, as well as the alligators at the bottom of his garden, he had once seen a rattlesnake on his drive, but it was no problem because a neighbour came round and battered it to death with a baseball bat. I was not reassured by this news.

He also told me there were two other snakes to keep a look out for. They were identical in that they had red, yellow and black markings on their back. But one was poisonous, one wasn't. They had a little saying to help you remember which was which, and it went something like 'if it's red then yellow he's a nice fellow, if it's black then red you'll end up dead'. One day I was in the gym in the garage and I was on the pec deck. All of a sudden this snake slithered towards me; it was black, yellow and red and, to be quite honest, I have no idea how I didn't shit myself.

I was trying to work out which type of snake it was. It slithered through the spokes in the wheels on my chair, up the machine I was working on and I was petrified.

I was shouting, 'Gouldie, Gouldie, GOULDIE!!!!!!'

He came in and asked me what was up.

I said, 'There's a fucking huge snake just gone behind me!'

He just picked it up nonchalantly, threw it in the garden and told me there was no reason to worry; it wasn't the poisonous kind.

You can imagine my relief!

We went to Corpus Christi in Texas for our next tournament and, after the last game, we went into a bar and had a contest to see who could drink the most 'Jaegermeister'. You had to drink five test tube shots to get a T-shirt. It was horrendous stuff and all the other lads wouldn't do it, but I told them to give it to me. Five minutes later I was on the floor, I was gone, but I got the T-shirt though!

Next we went to Houston for regionals. The Tampa Generals and the Storm could not enter the same region, so the Suncoast Storm was sent to play in the South Central region.

We had to come in the top two to qualify for Nationals, and getting the Storm to qualify was the main reason I was there. We played Houston, one of the favourites, in the semi-final. It was a close game but we ended up winning. So Tampa became the first franchise to send two teams to the National Championships.

Mission Accomplished.

In the regional final we played San Antonio and lost in triple overtime. My overriding memory is that one of the refs in the final was Terry Vinyard's girlfriend. She had made a harsh call on me right at the end of the game, which cost us the match. He went absolutely berserk at her and was screaming saying she was useless and that the relationship was over. It was absolutely hilarious. I didn't help matters by stirring it up, egging him on and telling him to give it to her.

She told him to fuck off, then turned to me and told me to fuck off as well. Still, I made the all-star team at that competition. For a Brit to go over and do that was quite an achievement. I am very proud of that.

Eventually we headed up to Boston for the Nationals. We played well and got to the semi-finals against Tennessee, but they had a great team and beat us easily. We then lost to Rick Draney's San Diego team in the 3rd/4th play off. Suncoast Storm came in 4th, but that was a huge achievement considering they were ranked 17th in the States when I got there.

At first I didn't feel homesick in Tampa but my sister-in-law had given birth to a baby, Matthew, five months earlier. He was my first nephew so I missed not seeing him.

However, getting an opportunity of living and playing in America, I didn't see the point in feeling homesick and I didn't allow myself to. Nobody had ever done what I was doing before and that excited me. Playing in the toughest league against the best players in the world was what I was all about. But as my time there was coming to an end I was ready to go home. I'd had enough. The constant training, flying and playing tournaments had taken its toll.

After we played in the Nationals in Boston the flight back to Tampa was delayed by six hours. Terry chose this time to ask me if I would come back the next year; my answer was, 'After six hours in this airport, no thanks!'

In fact, I was asked to go back to the States a year later. Connecticut wanted both Rob and I to sign for them as a package. That would have been a great laugh but we both had other issues in our lives at that time and we didn't go. A decision I think we both regret to this day. I certainly do.

THE GHOST AT GOULDIE'S

My last night in Tampa was very strange. I have never been so scared in my life. You can point a gun to my head and I wouldn't be as terrified as I was then. Generally I'm not frightened of anything. Put a snake in front of me, however, and I get the twitch on. Come at me with a needle, I'm nervous. This was something else though.

I flew back from Boston and was dropped off at Gouldie's house in the early hours. I had the place to myself as he had stayed on with his family in Boston. I started to get everything together to pack up for my flight home. It took me ages as I had so much stuff.

I went to bed quite early and was playing Tetris on my Game Boy. I dozed off. I woke up at 3 a.m. and could hear this music, UB40 doing their cover version of Elvis's 'I can't help falling in love with you'.

The music was getting louder and louder. Gouldie's house was a detached bungalow. I thought that maybe his neighbours were having a bit of a party. The song was almost deafening. I decided that I would have to go next door and tell them to turn it down as I had a long flight back home the next day. I went out of the bedroom into the kitchen, looked out and saw all the neighbours' lights were out. I turned round. Gouldie's bedroom light was on. This was not right as I was in the house alone. I remember thinking that there was someone in the house with me, so I went and got the biggest knife I could find in the kitchen.

Just picture it, a bloke in a wheelchair, stark naked with a foot long knife in his hand.

I just thought if there was someone in there, then they were going to get it before I did. I barged through the door fully expecting to see a burglar or some bloke with a beard and a banjo waiting to violate me.

There was absolutely nobody there.

But Gouldie's light was on. At the side of his bed was an alarm clock radio and the music was coming out of that.

The clock itself was flashing 12:00 but it was switched off!!!

I didn't know what was going on. To cap it all, his shower room light was also on. There was no reason for the radio to have come on; Gouldie always set his alarm for 8 a.m., and it was now just gone 3 a.m. even though the clock was flashing 12:00. To make it spookier it wasn't even switched on so it shouldn't have been doing anything anyway.

And who switched the lights on?

I couldn't turn the radio off because the switch was already in the off position, so I turned the volume down, switched the lights off, went back into my bedroom and locked the door. I went to bed with the knife in my hand and stayed awake till dawn.

I then got my stuff together and waited on the driveway for my lift to the airport to arrive at 8 a.m. There was no way I was staying in that house a moment longer than I had to. However, just like in the horror films, I went back into the house even though the audience was screaming, 'Don't!'

I needed another look before I left for the airport. I went into his bedroom only to find another mystery – the alarm clock was now switched on and showing the right time.

I thought to myself that it was really time to go home.

I explained all this to the lad who picked me up and he was spooked.

If someone told me the story I wouldn't believe it. I'm not into paranormal stuff at all. I like watching ghost programmes but I don't believe any of it. I was trying to think of a logical explanation for what had happened that night. But I couldn't find one.

I felt knackered on the flight home after not sleeping due to the paranormal alarm clock and lights. But I got no chance of kip because I was sat next to this Swedish bloke. He was a bit odd to look at. Out of the blue he asked me what my sexual preference was. I know it's like a scene out of a Swedish adult film but I'm not making it up.

I hadn't slept for a couple of days and, here I was sat next to a right weirdo. I told him I was into women.

He then told me that he worked at a mental hospital and dealt with men and women who were into animal pornography! A subject he began to talk about in graphic detail.

In the end I had to get the air stewardess to move him. On a long flight home the last thing you need is some weirdo go on about how to get jiggy with donkeys.

Once I was home, I waited a few days until I knew Gouldie would be back from Boston and gave him a call about the spooky goings on. He said that nothing like that had ever happened to him and all the electrics were fine. I'll be sat on my deathbed thinking about what really happened that night. Someone asked me if I was dreaming but I know I wasn't, as I had the knife in bed with me in the morning!

Rick Draney, *US Paralympian*

If I had to rate Mark as a rugby player when I first encountered him, I would say he was an above average player. In the early 90s rugby was really starting its growth in the US. Up until then, rugby was more of a 'fun' sport or recreational outlet – the chairs weren't very far along in their design/development, game strategy was somewhat limited due to a lack of knowledge/experience, there weren't as many teams, tournaments, or opportunities for 'serious' competition, and so on. Thus, a player with good athletic ability, determination, and good chair skills would stand out. I saw Mark as that type of individual. Personally, I never agreed (and still don't agree) with a 'foreigner' playing in the US QRA. I understood the reasoning and rationale behind it (back then, it was at least in part about helping to teach, promote, and grow the sport internationally – now, it's purely done by teams to try and win more games). So, in part, I viewed Mark at the Suncoast Storm as an unwelcome guest.

I had heard that one of the Florida rugby teams had a player from England that was pretty good, but honestly, I didn't give it too much thought back then. It wasn't until playing against him at Stoke Mandeville that I got a pretty good idea of who he was and what he was about as an athlete.

I didn't pay too much attention to rugby players or their reputations back then. Also, it was still relatively early in our competitive careers and I don't think that either of our reputations were then what they might be perceived now. I do remember hearing that he was 'a bit intense' but I sort of thought, 'Well, let's just see how intense he is.' At Stoke Mandeville, it was obvious that he competed with a lot of emotion and passion, to the point that he was obviously emotional losing to us, Team USA.

Chapter 6

Autonomic Dysreflexia

I learnt a lot about myself in Tampa, both as a person and a player. To be honest, before I went away I was already the best player in this country, but when I came back, I had gone up another few levels. It became very easy for me in the UK. I knew I could go out the night before a tournament, get blitzed and still get up and boss the show.

When I got back from Tampa though I had a break from rugby and me and my mate Jimmy partied big time. Later in the year we went to Tenerife.

Jimmy, *Mark's closest friend, remembers*

In 1994 we went to Tenerife and we had a competition, 'snog a dog'. Whoever won had their beer paid for the rest of that night. Eccy ended up snogging a girl who was the spitting image of Bet Lynch off Coronation Street.

God, she was ugly as it gets. She was that ugly we refused to pay up. Nobody in their right mind would suck face with someone that ugly but he did. It was a good laugh that holiday.

I hadn't seen my mates for a few months so the catching up was lively to say the least. Going out round St Helens at the time, there were only three pubs of note in the town centre along with one nightclub. That was probably the best social period of my life between 1994 and 1996. The lads and me got up to all kinds. One of our favourite tricks was when three of us would sit on a sofa in a pub with the wheelchair out in front of us. Everytime a girl would walk past we would ask them which one of us was the cripple. It was brilliant for me because they almost always got it wrong!

But between Nationals in June and the World Championships in August 1994, I suffered my first Autonomic Dysreflexia attack.

Today people with spinal cord injuries are educated about Autonomic Dysreflexia but nobody really discussed it with me after I was injured. Not long before the attack, I spoke to a basketball player who told me he had had an attack after ejaculating for the first time since his accident. I was totally fascinated by what he was saying.

One night, I was in the shower and suddenly I got an incredible pain in the back of my head and remembered the basketball player describing his pain. I immediately knew I had gone dysreflexic. Imagine the worst pain you ever had – and multiply it by 1,000. This was the most painful feeling I had ever experienced. I was clenching my teeth and screaming, tears were rolling down my face and I couldn't open my eyes.

Autonomic Dysreflexia is a condition where the blood pressure in a person with a spinal cord injury above T5–6 becomes excessively high. It is usually caused when a painful stimulus occurs below the level of the spinal cord injury.

The main causes of Autonomic Dysreflexia are related to problems with the bladder and bowel. Complications can become dangerous due to the fact that people cannot feel pain 'below' the level of their damage. So broken bones, pressure sores and in-growing toenails can trigger it. Over-stimulation during sexual activity to the pelvic region can also cause it.

A severe, untreated dysreflexia attack can lead to a stroke.

The on-call doctor came out to see me and gave me some painkillers, but they didn't help.

The additional problem I had was that I was to go down to Stoke Mandeville the very next day for the International Games, so I phoned a mate who'd had an attack like this before. He gave me some Nifedipine tablets.

Nifedipine tables are a necessity for anyone who is paralysed T6 and above. If a dysreflexia attack occurs, you have to place them under your tongue and bite them, and this will bring your blood pressure down.

When I got to Stoke, I went straight to Brian Worrall to explain the situation. He took me to the nurse and she did an ultra sound on my bladder. The ultra sound made everything clear. What had brought on the attack was that my bladder was retaining urine.

When my bladder contains around 500ml of urine it gives me the urge to go to the toilet. My bladder was retaining about 200ml, and it was causing me problems. I played the tournament, but every time I passed urine I got a pounding headache.

We got to the final again against America and again we lost but, at this point, I just wanted to get home and get the problem sorted. I was admitted to hospital and was taught to perform self-intermittent catheterisation. This enabled me to completely empty my bladder and that gradually solved the problem.

I was not too sure whether to put this experience on paper but Autonomic Dysreflexia is something that everybody should be aware of, especially anyone who has a spinal cord injury of T6 or above.

I have seen what it can do when it is severe.

A friend, who was on the National Championship winning Southport rugby team of 1992 with me, had a serious attack. When I went to see him he did not recognise me.

Autonomic Dysreflexia is a very, very serious issue. Especially to anyone T6 and above:

ALWAYS CARRY NIFEDIPINE!

Chapter 7

Lead up to Atlanta 1996

In 1995 I began to get very disillusioned with rugby, but I was convinced to play on after Brian phoned me and told me rugby had finally been let into the Paralympics.

I began training hard again in early 1996 as selection was in April and I really wanted to be in top shape. I got selected. There was never going to be any doubt, but it was still good to hear my name called out.

Later that year I went to the Nationals but I was carrying a shoulder injury. I asked if there was a physio at the tournament and someone told me that Cardiff had one. I went over to her and I do have to say she was extremely attractive, but I can also honestly add that giving her one was not at the top of my list of priorities.

I asked her politely if she would take a look at my shoulder.

'If you're going to chat me up you have to try harder than that,' she replied.

I looked at her in total disbelief and replied, 'Trust me, love, if I wanted to tap off with you I could, in fact, I would have had you out in the car park by now.'

I went away fuming and couldn't believe what she had just said.

Cardiff had a 3-point player who thought he was better than me and that he should have been picked for Atlanta. I didn't like him, and the feeling was mutual. It soon got back to me that he had been telling people that I'd tried it on with the physio, so I decided that I was going to target him and outplay all the other Cardiff players. He wasn't so gobby when I started pushing backwards with the ball on my knee, which left him chasing after me rather pathetically.

Now I am sorry, but if someone pushing backwards can go faster than you are pushing forwards, then you need to stop having delusions of grandeur immediately.

THE PHYSIO LOVELY

At another point during the game, I was trapped on the sideline right next to the Cardiff bench where our lovely physio friend sat. As I was bouncing the ball, I turned to her and said, 'I'm going to flip this ball over their heads, go around them and score but, before I do, I want you to tell me how good I am.'

'You are good but you're also an arrogant little shit,' she answered. At which point I did exactly what I said I was going to do.

In my humble opinion, a lot of people confuse arrogance with confidence; those that do generally don't have the ability to do what they say they are going to do, or just haven't got a clue what they are talking about. Granted, I have just demonstrated I can be arrogant when I want to be, but only if someone has annoyed me or shown disrespect. If our friend the physio had not been so rude and obnoxious to me, then everything would have been fine, and we would just have had a good, clean, hard game.

In the lead up to Atlanta 96, I got involved with a girl and, believe me, she is a book in her own right. Jimmy and me used to go out into St Helens town centre every Thursday night. We were in a nightclub where it was a pound a bottle so you could get hammered quite cheaply. I noticed this girl staring at me. She looked dirty and I don't mean as in she needed a wash. She had a mate with her who, to put it politely, had prominent teeth.

The pair of them came over and started talking to us.

She told me she had seen me earlier in the night and that, when she first saw me, she thought I had just been sat down.

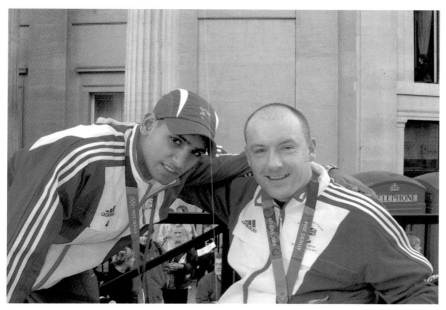

With Amir Khan, fellow Olympian.

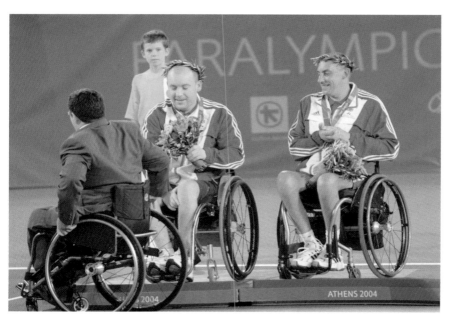

Olympic medallist.

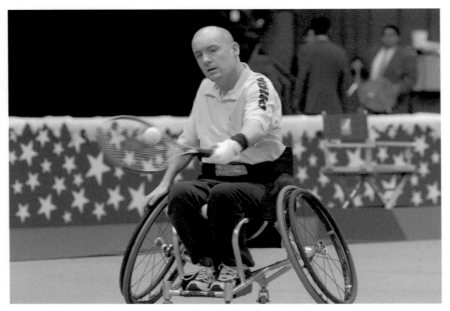

In play.

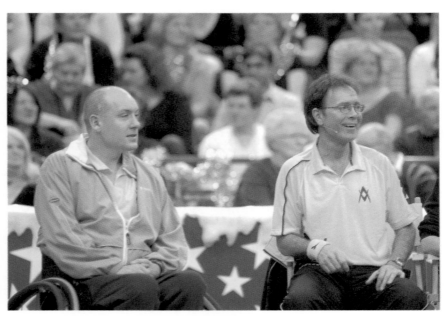

'Congratulations' – at the Cliff Richard Foundation.

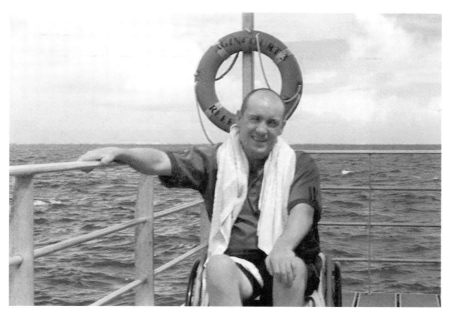

All at sea.

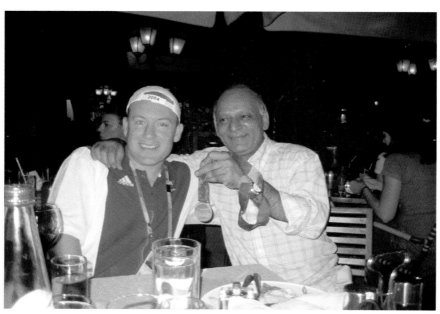

With Dr Soni, who treated me when I broke my neck.

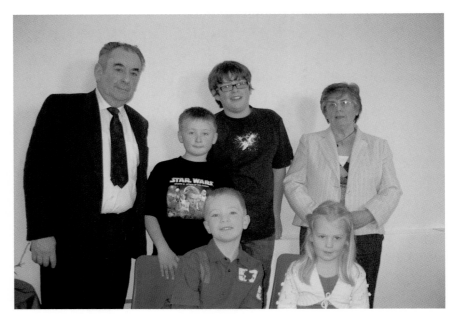

Mum and Dad.

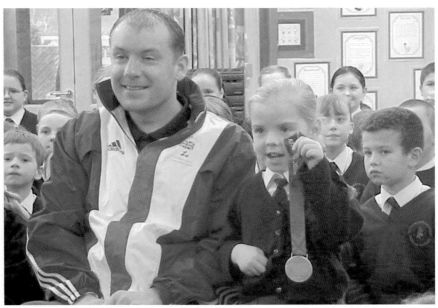

Kids love seeing the medal.

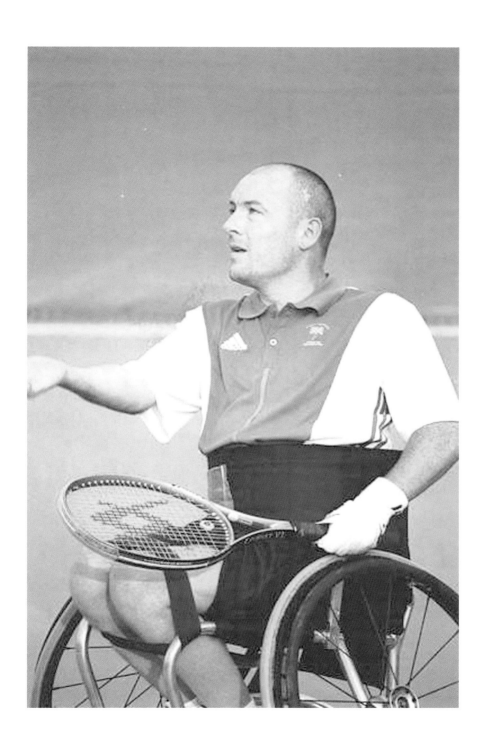

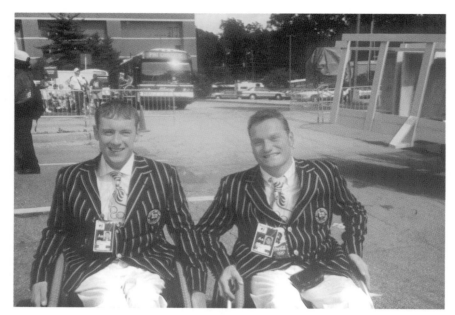

Me and Rob, Atlanta 1996.

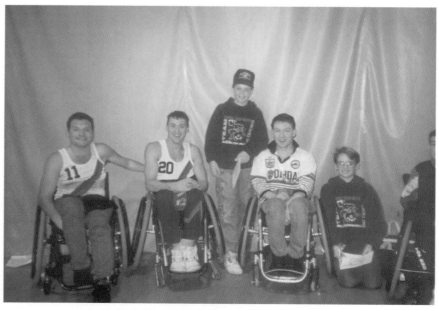

L-R: Rob Tarr, Keith Jones, me, Toronto 1993.

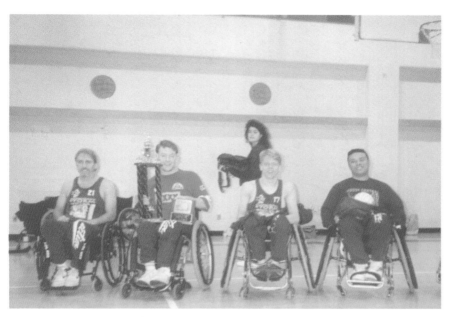

Regionals in Houston. Suncoast Storm, 2004.

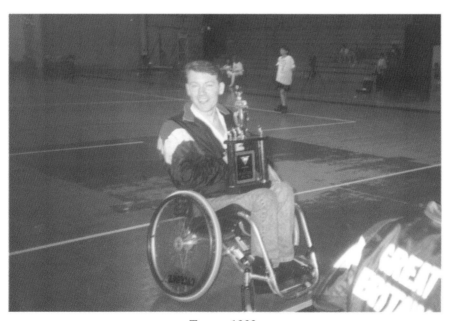

Tampa 1993.

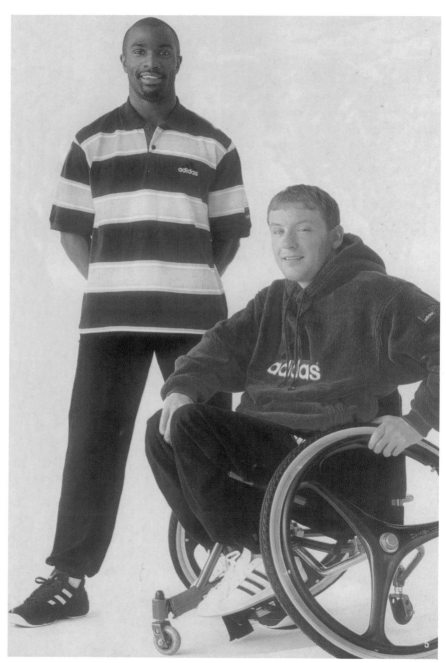

Derek Redmond and me, advertising.

'I am,' I said.

She had told her mate that I had really nice eyes; then she stood up and noticed that I was in a wheelchair. I asked if that bothered her and she said it didn't.

Eventually, we would meet up every Thursday in town. We nicknamed her mate 'Ken Dodd' because, although she had a good body and a lovely personality, bless her, her teeth were something else. The thing was, we would call her Ken Dodd to her face and she just never clicked. A mate of mine started to go out with her, so to make up a cosy foursome, I started seeing her mate. However it turned out she was living with a bloke who people kept telling me was a bit of a psycho.

She would tell me that he was knocking her about and so on. It got to the point where wherever I was in town, he would be there glaring at me. One morning all the tyres on her car had been slashed. At first we thought Ken Dodd had been trying to blow them up with her teeth, but we quickly arrived at the conclusion that the psycho had paid a visit.

It was one of those relationships where we were always arguing. True to form, I would later find out that she was literally 'the good-time girl'.

When we were out in a nightclub, she would be flirting with lads to wind me up. This would annoy my mates more than me and they got a bit protective. I found the whole thing fascinating though as it had this element of danger.

It started getting nasty though. Her ex came up to me and said, 'You don't want to go out with her. She'll only cause you trouble.'

I didn't listen though and, then, she invited me on her works party. There was a lad she worked with in the pub, a lad who she had told me had kept asking her out. He stood on a table and starting singing the Kate Bush song 'Running up that Hill', while looking at me with a big grin on his face. I was furious about that. He then proceeded to take a mouthful of beer and spray it over me. I told her I was leaving, as what he had done was bang out of order. And that he should apologise or else.

SATURDAY NIGHT FEVER

The next Saturday I was in the nightclub and all her workmates were in there too, including the beer-spraying lad. My mates were gunning for him because of what he had done. She was on the dance floor with him and they started kissing. I didn't see it but one of my mates did and he went straight over and smacked him straight across the dance floor. The lad went skidding right past me, seemingly in slow motion like something out of Tom and Jerry. Then he got up and legged it.

I didn't see the girl for a couple of days after that. Then, two days before I was due to go to Atlanta, she rang me; she gave me a letter telling me that I shouldn't open it until I was on the plane over to the States. By this time, I'd had enough and had only gone to her house to pick up a video camera that I was borrowing from Ken Dodd.

On the plane to the States, I was sat next to Rob Tarr and he opened the letter. He began howling with laughter. She said she was madly in love with me and was going to sell her house to buy a bungalow for us. It had become a huge joke by this point. In the weeks leading up to this there had always been a red car parked outside her house. I asked who it belonged to and was told that it was next door's. I didn't think much of it. However, I later found out it belonged to the lad who spat the beer on me.

By the time I got back from Atlanta, she had moved him in! This was three weeks after she wrote she was buying a bungalow for us.

I certainly knew how to pick them – back then.

The whole episode meant I didn't have a very good opinion of women at the time. However, my opinion and attitude changed when I met Lucy.

All this drama went on during my preparation for Atlanta but it certainly didn't affect my playing, as I was voted Great Britain's best player and received a certificate from the Paralympic Organising Committee congratulating me on my outstanding performance.

A couple of years later bungalow bird phoned and asked if she could see me. When I went to meet her, she got out of the car with a baby!

Mentally I got the calculator out and started to panic. She told me to relax as it wasn't mine and she just wanted to see how I was. It was bizarre. I wanted to know what she wanted and she told me she just wanted to see me.

I listened to what she had to say and I could not believe what I was hearing. I never thought anything this girl could do would surprise me but this certainly did. After our relationship and all the problems she caused me, I disliked her but, after hearing what she told me, I ended up feeling sorry for her. She obviously had issues and she has to live with what she told me for the rest of her life.

Chapter 8

Atlanta – Mark and Rob's Excellent Adventure

The lead up to Atlanta was great. The event itself was terrible. In the week before it started we worked out at a big naval base in Pensacola and that was fantastic. Brian Worrall told us there was no leaving the base, but he allowed Rob and me our usual bit of freedom and the pair of us headed off at night into the Spanish quarter. Brian had the sense to do stuff that wasn't in the handbook. I can't help wondering if there wasn't some connection between the fact that he would turn the odd blind eye to some of Rob's antics and mine – and how well we played for him.

At the base after training one day, there was a group of black lads on the sidelines. We got talking to them. One of them was Roy Jones Jnr, one of the best boxers of all time. Jones was from Pensacola and apparently could have been a professional basketball player. It was a great experience meeting him. I got him to sign my T-shirt but one of the support staff with our team washed it and so washed off the autograph.

The Mayor of Pensacola invited the Great Britain team down to an official function. I didn't want to go and I wasn't wrong. We were put on a table with a group of athletes from another sport. One of them was spitting whilst eating and it put us off our food slightly. It certainly wasn't the reason we left but it was the straw that broke the camel's back you might say. We told Brian we were going and we got a taxi and headed into town.

When the training camp finished, we had to get on coaches for the drive to Atlanta. This was a 7-hour bus ride and our driver was this hillbilly American who had that 'yawl' accent, a mullet hair cut and a rather sad 1970s porno moustache.

He decided to put a video on for us. However, this was no ordinary video, this was something akin to 'when pets go wrong' or 'fireworks – delicious but deadly' that you see on Channel 5 but a lot more gory!!

Amongst the footage it showed was a bomb disposal guy getting his head blown off. I sat back in my seat and thought how many more hours of this?

'I've got more of these if you want to watch them,' he said.

'Just the one will do, thanks,' I said.

Seven hours on a coach with a bunch of people in wheelchairs is not my idea of fun. Surprisingly for America, the coaches did not have lifts and so it took ages to get everyone on. A coach holds about 40 people and some muppet in their immense wisdom decided that all the wheelchairs were getting on the same one. Have you got any idea how long it takes to lift 40 athletes in wheelchairs on the same coach? It's an absolute bloody nightmare.

The majority of the party had to be carried on – and that included Rob. It wasn't just the rugby team; there were a number of other sports as well.

It took about three hours to get everyone aboard. If you were first on, it meant three hours of sitting there doing nothing so Rob and me hid, in order to go on last. This proved to be a very good move because it was last on – first off. As soon as the coach stopped in Atlanta, we were off like a shot.

Then we had to go through accreditation. Accreditation at a Paralympics is one long queue where you have your photo taken, your pass made up and you fill in a number of forms declaring that you have never been to a terrorist training camp in Uzbekistan and that it is not your intention to shoot the President of the United States, although ... now you mention it.

CHATTING UP THE CHINA BIRD

We had a lovely Chinese girl seeing to us – not literally. Rob and I hit her with all the best chat up lines we could muster but she was having none of it. She told us she had been there all day and plenty of others had already tried, so we were wasting our time. However, true to form, later in the tournament, one of us ended up cracking what was originally a tough nut.

Once in the Olympic village it was down to business. Our first training session meant another coach journey. However, the driver, after cruising round for a bit, admitted he didn't know where to go and took us back to the village. It was a shambles.

Christopher Reeve, who had played Superman before an accident paralysed him, addressed the stadium at the opening ceremony as did the US Vice-President Al Gore. As with any event like this where VIPs give speeches, it was the usual 'courage, great to have you here, aren't you really wonderful people' – lines that I've heard a million times before and a million times since.

There were performances from Hall & Oates and Carly Simon.

When we got to the accommodation though, things went downhill quicker than a blind, pissed slalom skier. The conditions in the Olympic village at Georgia Tech were disgraceful. It was dirty and the rooms were so small it was untrue. Rob and I made a video of our time there; it is hilarious and entitled 'Rob and Mark's Excellent Adventure'.

Eight of us shared the same apartment; it got heated at times as we were in such a cramped space. It caused a bit of bitching so Rob and me would get back from the training sessions and go out. We just used to say that we had been to the bar on the site. The truth was we needed time away from some people in the apartment.

The room Rob and I shared was so small that if I wanted to get out of the bed I had to push Rob's chair out of the room. Did I complain? Too right I did!

Everybody in the whole village complained. Even the athletes from countries who take a dump in holes in the floor and live in dreadful conditions complained. The beds and walls were filthy. To get to the food hall in the village took a 20-minute push up the biggest hill in the world and, when you eventually got there, the food was crap.

It was a poor effort on the organisers' part. I wanted to go and stay in a hotel but no one was allowed to leave the village, as security was tight. Only a few weeks before, a bomb had gone off at the Olympics, and an unfortunate security guard was wrongly accused of planting it so he could play the hero. As a result, you had to go through X-ray machines and other checks to enter the village. I knew the conditions were going to send me crazy. Brian wisely picked up on this and gave Rob and me the usual leeway; we could have our nights out as long as we didn't let him down.

We went out of the campus and a security guard told us that if we pushed up the big hill there was a great bar called Billy Bobs. The manager, a Mexican bloke called Angel, served us. I told him we would be coming in regularly and wanted a quiet spot in the corner where no one would bother us. He started talking to us and gave us a menu that listed around a hundred different beers. He said that before we left Atlanta he wanted us to have tried every single one of them and they would all be free of charge. We asked for his biggest bowl of chicken wings and started working our way through the beers. Every night we were in there and every night we drank for free. All he asked in return was a signed T-shirt, as it was a sports bar and he wanted it for the wall.

A fair trade, I thought.

ONE HUNDRED FINE BEERS – ONE FINE TRY

It kicked off one night though. We'd had a couple of beers in Billy Bobs. The next morning Brian stormed into our apartment going berserk and asking, 'Where's Mark and Rob?' We didn't know what was up. He asked us how many beers we had had

90

the night before. We told him we'd only had a couple. He said, 'We're in trouble now, with you two fighting in there.'

We didn't have a clue what he was on about. He was shouting about us letting him down.

I asked him what the score was. He said there had been trouble in Billy Bobs and we had been seen in there. I told him that we hadn't noticed any trouble. The Chef de Mission, who is the head of the whole Paralympic team, came in.

Seeing him, I realised it was being treated as a serious matter.

The story was that a couple of athletes from another country had kicked off in the bar and a couple of the British rugby team had been seen in there. Someone put two and two together and came up with Rob and me. In fact, I later found out it had happened an hour after we had left.

We thought it best to lay low and away from Angel's 100 brands of beer for a bit but were soon back in Billy Bobs. Our new best friend, Angel, treated us as long lost sons, and served us first, no matter how long the queue.

As for the on court action, our quarter-final match was against Australia. We were 5 points down with 2 minutes to go.

It looked like an impossible task as we were so far behind. As the captain, I told the others on court that we were the only four that could get us out of this, as we couldn't rely on any of the other players on the bench. I also said that this was the only chance we were going to have, so we had to dig in deep or else we were going home.

Somehow we managed to claw it back, and with about 10 seconds remaining, the scores were level. The Aussies had possession and were heading for goal. If they had scored, it would have been game over, with us knocked out of the Paralympic games. They had this big lad they called 'the Truck' who was huge and he was heading for goal. I was chasing after him, when all of a sudden, Rob came from nowhere and cleaned him out. The ball flew up in the air on our line and almost in slow motion, Rob knocked the ball to me and shouted, 'Now fuck off!'

I spun round and looked up at the clock. There were 8.2

seconds remaining. Now the fastest I had ever gone from one side of the court to the other was just over 7 seconds but don't forget, this was at the end of a very gruelling game. I put my head down and went for it.

You're only allowed 10 seconds before you have to bounce the ball or pass it. With less than 10 seconds on the clock I knew my only hope was to put the ball on my knee and go for it. I kept expecting the bell to go before I got to the line, but it didn't. I scored. I looked up at the clock and there were 2.2 seconds to go. I had done it in 6 seconds. Everyone was going mad on our bench.

I just went past the Aussie bench, grinning at them, screaming, 'How good was that?'

They had 2.2 seconds left on the clock. With wheelchair rugby the clock only starts running when someone touches the ball. 'The Truck' was down by our line. It was clear that the Aussies were going to try and launch it to him. Their in-bounder threw it but he couldn't have done a worse job if he had tried, as it landed right on my knee!

I simply held the ball above my head, looking to our bench, nodding 'game over'. The Aussies were going mad at me. The ref blew the final whistle.

Pandemonium!

I have never seen anything like it, people were going wild, and everyone dove in on me. It was one of the most memorable, special moments in my sporting career. Loads of kids were asking for my autograph. Nobody could quite believe what had just happened.

Sometimes I can't believe that dramatic finish really happened, so it's good to have Rob's memories.

Rob Tarr *says*

The quarter final against Australia in Atlanta will always live in the memory for Mark's last second winner. I tackled one of their players, flicked the ball to Mark and gave him the instruction to 'fuck off'. I kept looking up at the clock, as he headed to the other end, 5–4–3, he was there.

Unbelievable.

It was talked about for the rest of the tournament. The Australians still talk about it now. It was a Hollywood ending.

After the Australia game I was brought back down to earth when an official told me I was required for a drugs test. Drugs tests are a nuisance because you've got some bloke watching you go the toilet. You are allowed to take someone with you so I took Brian along.

One of the Aussies was being tested too. Brian and I were ripping him to bits.

It took ages for me to 'go'. In the end five cans of Coke did the trick. The game had finished at 10.30 p.m., we only got out of there about 1 a.m. On the way back I got talking to a female wheelchair rugby official, who somehow managed to smuggle herself into the village, much to Rob's delight.

Back in the village, at about 2 a.m., I was still buzzing from the end of the game plus the caffeine injection of five cans of coke.

I couldn't sleep so woke Rob up and we went round the village for a bit.

It was so surreal because one of the security guards was chatting to a volunteer and they were talking about the rugby match between Great Britain and Australia. They didn't know who we were and were going on about this kid for Great Britain who had scored in the very last second.

We pretended we didn't know what they were talking about but I was buzzing inside. It was quite funny.

An American tennis player called Kev Whalen, who I have great respect for, was there that night. Frequently at tennis tournaments we've been at together, he brings the Australia match up. He's a real sports buff and still insists that what I did that night is one of the greatest sporting moments he's ever seen. Well I'm not going to contradict him. I just wish I could track the video down!

OF BEERS AND BEDS

One of the best laughs we had was when Rob and me went into Atlanta and had a few beers; we got back to the apartment and Rob tried to transfer onto the bed – but due to the substantial amount of alcohol he consumed he missed and fell asleep on the floor. He didn't awake till 3 p.m. the next day.

This meant that because the room was so small neither did I. One night, he came in drunk and I sprayed shaving foam all over his face. He woke up wanting to know who had done it but was so drunk that all you could hear were mumbles, mixed with a few expletives. I filmed it and on the video you can see a bed, a wheelchair and a whacked out cripple with shaving foam all over his face.

Another day we got back to the room and there was Rob, lying on his front naked with a flag sticking out of his arse, singing 'God save the Queen'. Patriotism Rob-style.

The semi-final was against the USA. They were coached by Terry Vinyard and had Joe and Goldie from Tampa in their team. They were just too powerful for us and we got well and truly beat. Physically I was feeling it by this point, as I had to do more than my fair share in the earlier matches. I had now come to expect that in all our matches I would have two players marking me and as a result it got more and more difficult for me. We had a string of hard games as we'd lost our first game against the Canadians. Rob and I didn't start that game, as Brian selected a big lad called Roy in the hope that he would win a lot of ball; then we could come on later and do our stuff. Roy had no trouble winning the ball but didn't have a clue what to do with it. The best example of this was when he sped off with the ball down the court ... the wrong way and scored a cracker in his own goal.

We were all shouting 'Roy? Roy? ROY?' He never played again after that. By the time Rob and I got on the court, we were 6 behind and it was just too big of a gap to make up.

The bronze medal play off was against New Zealand. They had a very strong team and they were like a bunch of pitbulls.

Before the game they did the Haka routine. We had this big lad called Jenks with a bald head and we painted his face white and his tongue jet black. We made him sit directly in front of the guy leading the Haka and stick his black tongue out at him. Everyone was dying laughing, including a couple of the Kiwis.

The New Zealanders had done their homework and targeted me, giving me a tough time all game. They had one small lad who we called Oddjob because his head was the same size as his body and he was the spitting image of the Bond villain. I was clean through on goal and 'Oddjob' caught my back wheel, which sent me spinning out of my chair. I got back in my chair and lost it. I went straight for him. Suddenly I was surrounded by his team-mates; unfortunately my back up didn't arrive.

New Zealand were a niggly, aggressive team but also well drilled and skillful. Rob and I stood up to them but I felt the others didn't have the stomach for the fight. We lost by 9 points and I was gutted. As we came off court, we were signing autographs and I threw my shirts to a couple of kids in wheelchairs. I signed a ball for Trey, a referee I had known from my Tampa days.

But it was one of those moments. As soon as the final hooter went I knew that I would never play a game of rugby again. When Brian came on court, I said, 'That's it, I am done.'

On the way back to our changing room, we had to pass the New Zealand changing room. It had been a good battle and I think they respected me for fronting up to them. I also knew I'd never play another game of rugby, so I decided to go into their room. I went in and one of them said, 'Whoa, look who's here.' I immediately got the impression I was not welcome.

I said, 'Look, I've come in to say I'm retiring, congratulations you deserve your bronze medal.' They surprised me and said, 'We feel for you mate, do you want a drink?'

I went and got Rob. An hour later we were still in their dressing room!

I believe Brian feels let down by certain things that went on at the Atlanta Paralympics.

We were good enough to have won a medal. Yet we finished

fourth. We let Brian down. We had come second in the International Games previous to Atlanta and, while America were streets ahead of everybody, we had beaten Canada who was considered the second best team in the world. There were players on the Great Britain side who, when push came to shove, bottled it. I genuinely thought our starting team were good enough to have left Atlanta with a medal, but unfortunately the bench was too weak and this is probably the reason why we never did.

Brian has a lot of insight into the reasons we didn't do as well as I feel we should have done.

He is no longer involved in wheelchair rugby.

Brian Worrall, *coach*

Many things weren't ideal in Atlanta, the heat for one. The team played well, apart from a couple of them and that was down to the heat. It was a real shame we didn't get in the medals. I think Mark was disappointed with how a number of players performed. I don't think he understood that this was down to the heat.

He was definitely the best rugby player in this country. When he went to play tennis, I was disappointed but I can understand why he did it. I had made a similar decision when I had to choose between swimming (at which I'd won a medal) and rugby myself. If he'd have stuck with the rugby, who knows how good he could have become? Mark would have been good at any sport he chose.

As for a funny story about Mark, I don't think I have any that could be put in a book!

He was a bit of a one for the ladies, put it that way.

Rugby was like a brotherhood. Having been a soldier you were close to the people you fought with and I would put Mark amongst those men. Rob was another one; they were a pleasure to work with, although over the years memories maybe become a lot rosier!

BACK TO THE WALL

In the pressure situation, when your back is against the wall, the top players thrive. I know myself that when my back is against the wall and someone thinks they have me beat, I rise to the challenge. To be honest, I hadn't really wanted to play wheelchair rugby anymore prior to Atlanta. I had started playing my tennis, but Brian persuaded me, saying that wheelchair rugby had finally gained acceptance as a Paralympic event.

The memories I took away from the 1996 Atlanta Paralympics were that the organisation was a big letdown but with Rob around the event certainly had its moments, as my mum and dad remember –

Pat

Mark lost out on a medal in Atlanta and that's why he took up tennis, he wanted to rely on himself.

Jimmy

The one thing he did get at Atlanta, though, was to be given the freedom of Pensacola.

To give a flavour of our off the field and, you may think, off the wall adventures in Atlanta, I'd like to include an extract from a video we made which we call

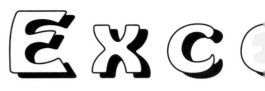

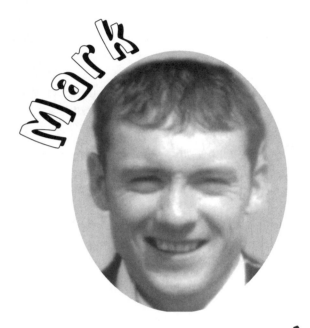

No holds barred
All birds bared
No bars missed

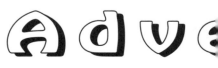

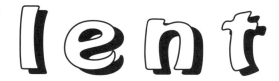

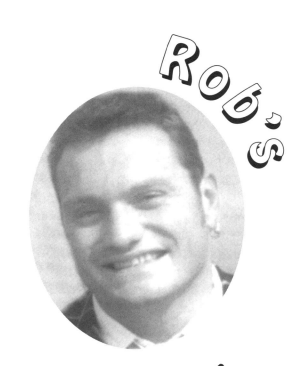

'Disturbing'
'Disturbed'

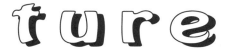

MARK: The stars of this highly disturbing and thought provoking documentary are Rob Tarr.

ROB: How you all doing there? And starring Mark Eccleston.

MARK: And here you have Robbie Tarr's bed.

Rob bounces up and down on the specially adapted bed for the 'disabled'

ROB: This bed is going to be taking some hammer.

Cut to a few days later

MARK: We've now been here five days and Rob Tarr is still in bed.

ROB: Are you zooming up my arse again? I'm sure you're bent.

Mark zooms in on a large plaster stuck to Rob's arse

MARK: What's that on your arse?

ROB: It's Granuflex, I got a friction burn shagging.

MARK: Here is Rob with four items of mail. There may not seem anything curious about that but all four are from the same bird, posted on the same day. Here with an adaptation is Rob.

Rob reads a letter

ROB: 'I long to feel the heat from your thighs, I love it when you make love to me, all of our lovemaking is special'.

MARK: This girl is sick, how long have you been seeing her?

ROB: 3 weeks.

Cut to the room at night and Roy is in bed

ROB: This is our friend Roy.

MARK: It's one o'clock in the morning and we've just put a huge frog in his bed. We can't find it so we are going to debag him.

Rob is now trying to take off Roy's urine leg bag

Cut to outside the bedroom in the sun. Mark and Rob who are dressed in the less than flattering GB Team suits with the rest of the squad sat around

ROB: Here we have Mr Mark Eccleston, what are you doing here at the Paralympics?

MARK: Being pissed around, messed about, we were supposed to be going to a Government function by bus but the buses didn't even know we were going. So we have been sat out in the sun baking whilst looking like ice cream men; we are now not going the function and are going to go to the pub instead.

ROB: Are we going on the piss?

MARK: Yes. And here we have Mr Rob Tarr, can you explain why you are dressed as an ice cream man?

ROB Well there was a cricket match and Dickie Bird wasn't there and I was asked to do some bowling.

MARK And your figures were?

ROB 36–24–44.

Any impression that we had sex on the brain is false and I will sue for defamation

ROB: We're going to Buckhead where they sell lots of Budweiser.

Cut to very cramped room in Paralympic village

ROB: Welcome to the penthouse suite. Plenty of room, and quite luxurious. Here is my bed and just look at the coke stains.

MARK: Are you sure they are coke stains and you've not pissed yourself? Anyway, you are sharing this room with Mark Eccleston, is there enough room?

ROB: Here's Mark's bed and here's my bed.

MARK: So anytime Mark wants to leave the room you have to get out too because it's so cramped.

ROB: I woke up this morning thinking I was having my penis washed and it was actually Mark washing his penis.

There now follows what the film trade calls a radical cut to Mark and Rob as they enter the stadium with the rest of the GB athletes as part of the opening ceremony

Music plays and dancers appear

MARK: Rob, what do you think of that blonde there?

Cut to then US Vice-President Al Gore as he finishes a welcoming address

MARK: Bullshit!

Cut to the Kiwi team doing the Haka on court, then back to Mark and Rob after the match

MARK: OK, Rob, we've just played New Zealand and got beat, how do you feel?

ROB: To sum it up in one word, shit.

Cut to a shot of a very steep hill

MARK: Now this is the hill that you have to push all the way up if you want something to eat. When you've been out on the booze like Rob here and you're absolutely bladdered, it's not very nice.

ROB: No, I don't feel very well at all.

MARK: Can you tell us what time you got in this morning, Mr Tarr?

ROB: Well I would estimate around 5 or 6 a.m. but I'm not sure, as I can't remember anything after 1 a.m.

MARK: Can you tell us why you slept on the floor and only got up at 3 in the afternoon?

ROB: I misjudged my transfer when I came in, missed the bed completely and fell on the floor.

MARK: Did you get undressed?

ROB: No, these are the clothes I had on last night.

MARK: You scruff.

Cut to Rob in the shower

MARK: What are you doing Rob? Hurry up; I'm dying for a piss.

ROB: I'm washing my winkle.

Rob sprays Mark with water

MARK: You bastard.

Cut to bedroom. I have replaced Rob's liberal use of the f-word with the word 'duck'

MARK: We have just got in and it's 8.30 in the morning and Rob Tarr is dead and snoring like a herd of bull elephants. I have sprayed shaving foam all over his face and he still hasn't woken up, shocking. Rob are you getting up now?

ROB: Duck off!

MARK: Are you getting up?

ROB: (Incomprehensible.)

MARK: Come on Rob.

ROB: Duck off.

MARK: Smile for the camera Robbie.

ROB: Who ducking shaving foamed me? Duck off you, Duck off you ... duck.

MARK: Time to get up Rob.

ROB: Duck off who's ducking shaving foamed me? Ducking

MARK: No idea Rob.

ROB: It's you, you bastard. Duck, ducking bastard it's ducking you.

MARK: So are you getting up or what?

ROB: DUCK OFF.

**Cut to inside of stadium, closing ceremony starts, cut to shot
of dancers doing the Macarena. Mark is filming and as he
pans round sees Rob pointing at one particular dancer with
a nice bottom, both Rob and camera zoom in. Cue the
credits and end music.**

PRACTICAL JOKES

A lot of things happened with the rugby tours with Rob and me
playing practical jokes on each other. On one tour, I owed him
one big time. We had all been on a night out and were pushing
back to the hotel. One player was so drunk he fell out of his
wheelchair and he couldn't get back in.

All of a sudden, this car stopped and two gorgeous women got
out. They helped him back into his chair and then one of them
came over to me, started chatting and asked if we needed any
escorts. I said we were fine as we had plenty of physios with us.

She then made it clear she was a very different type of escort.
Rob was out of earshot so I gave the two girls his room number
at the hotel and said for them to be there in ten minutes.

Another time, Rob and I had been up to shenanigans in the
social club. I crept back into the dormitory we shared at 3 a.m.,
as quietly as possible so as not to wake anyone up, especially
not Brian. Only for Rob to come bounding in five minutes later,
shaking Brian's bed and shouting. 'GUESS WHAT WE'VE JUST
BEEN DOING!'

Nice one Rob.

Rob Tarr

*Mark and I were a double act, and we would always room together.
He was a very, very good player. However he didn't like being let
down by the team. Everything that Mark did he gave 100%.*

*He fell out with a few team members that he didn't feel were pulling
their weight.*

*I'm glad I starred in 'Rob and Mark's Excellent Adventure'. Having
played in so many tournaments, they all seem to merge into one and*

this was a good way of sorting out the memories. Forget about the rugby, this was all about the exploits that we got up to.

The conditions in Atlanta weren't great. Mark and me were in a little box room. It was so small that I had to get my chair out of the room before Mark could get out. There would be nights where I would come in drunk at about 7 or 8 a.m. and pass out till 3 p.m., meaning Mark would have to wait till then before he could leave the room. We had a very good time though.

The more you tell Mark he can't do something the more determined he is to prove you wrong. I think he missed the camaraderie of the rugby lot though. I think the tennis was a bit of a lonely time for him. I don't think he ever really made a friend in the tennis community like he had with me. He had a fantastic career on the net. Full credit to him, he did incredibly well.

I know Mark went on to become the World's Number 1 in Tennis, but I also know that he missed his days as a Rugby Player.

MURDERBALL

In late 2005, a film was released about wheelchair rugby entitled 'Murderball' which played up the brutal nature of the sport. When I played it wasn't so bad, there was a bit of chair contact, but the chairs we used were like standard basketball chairs. The game allowed anyone who had a bit of talent to play with skill and flair. Now it's stupid, it's more like 'Robot Wars' with metal bars coming out everywhere. The chairs look more like dodgem cars and it's just a game of block. There are no players left who can dummy or pass a great ball. It's got to the stage where I watch it and view it as 'crash bang wallop'. There is a lot of chair contact and the chairs do get messed up. It wasn't as bad in my day. Now you can have a low point player taking a high point player out because he has a chair with hooks on it.

The rugby days were fantastic. Rugby had the camaraderie. I found it was a lot more relaxed and, with it being a team thing, you struck up good relationships. The craic that Rob and me had and the relationship we had with Brian ... it was all very, very special.

Chapter 9

Rugby, Clock Face Style

When I came back from Atlanta in September 1996, I decided to have a break. It was like a massive release valve. I was gutted that we had come fourth in the rugby, but relieved that the previous ten months had come to an end. All the training and hassle was over. I had made the decision that I was packing in the rugby, and that I was going to chill out until January.

I still did a little light training, but for the most part, I was deciding what to do next.

I went out a lot around St Helens at this time and had some very interesting encounters.

The disabled toilets in one particular nightclub didn't have a lock on the door. Everyone used to go in there, which annoyed me a fair bit. One night I was bursting to go to the toilet and I went in; inside was a lad and a girl I knew and they were having full on sex. I looked at them, expecting them to leave. Leave they did not, so I just told them to move over so I could have a burst.

They didn't stop!

As the woman was panting and moaning in the throes of passion, she somehow managed to say, 'Hiya, Eccy, how are you mate? How's the rugby going?'

'I've packed it in,' came my somewhat bemused reply.

Then the lad joined in with a breathless, 'Yeah, yeah, he's playing tennis now.'

There was a full five-minute three-way conversation going on as they were going at it good style and, impressively, they never once broke stride. That was probably one of the most memorable toilet breaks I've ever had, but I did leave before the grand finale.

Around this time a thoroughly enjoyable part of my life began. I started to coach an 'able-bodied' junior rugby league team.

Clock Face had an under-15s team, and they were struggling. They were at the bottom of the league and in front of the disciplinary committee all the time for fighting. My old mate Moff said that he had been asked to coach the side. He agreed on one condition – that I did it with him. My first reaction was to say I couldn't do it. People then started badgering. I was very apprehensive but thought that I might as well give it a go. So I did. It had always been in the back of my mind to get involved with a rugby team somehow.

Moff told me when the next training session was, and said that he would introduce me to the team and that I could say a few words. I have played in six world championship finals and the Paralympics, and yet I've never been so nervous in my life, knowing that I had to go into a dressing room with twenty little psychos and give a talk. These kids were the type that would have the police come down to matches and watch them.

I looked round the dressing room and, to my huge relief, they were as good as gold. They listened to every word I said. I told them that I knew what it took to win and that I believed I could help them improve.

They were well up for it and we started from there.

Some of the team remember that first meeting:

Mark Heesome

The first thing I noticed about Mark when he entered the Clock Face dressing room was obviously the fact that he was in a wheelchair. The other thing was how powerful he was.

When he spoke we listened. He just came across as a very wise man. He was the type of man you listened to.

Adam Langley

I was Mark's mum and dad's paperboy so I knew him. I remember very well when he turned up to coach us at Clock Face. The team was really struggling at the time. It sounds a bit bad looking back but when he first came in and we saw him in a wheelchair, we didn't take him seriously. That soon changed though. He gave us a 20 minute speech and it was incredible. He's a really good talker and he was even better as a coach, he was fantastic.

Ian Moffatt

I coached Clock Face junior rugby league side with Eccy. I was the feet on the pitch and he was the brains off the pitch. Eccy used to tell the kids, on a regular basis, that he was ten times better than me!

The team was shocking when we took over. It was the gap Mark was looking for though. It kept him involved on the rugby side of things. He could explain things to people very easily. He came up with different moves for the side and you wouldn't believe the turn around in the team. We gave them the strength to believe in themselves. They sometimes believed in themselves a little too much and enjoyed the odd barny even more than we did. It was one in, all in!

When I was coaching with him, if there was a player who wasn't up to scratch I would lose patience with them. Eccy wouldn't; he had time for them all.

TACKLES AND NIGGLES

My first impression was that if they got it together, they could be a good team. They had some great little players on the side. They lost the first match narrowly to Halton Hornets but I felt the only reason they lost was that they weren't fit enough. I knew we could get that sorted.

Our next match was against Bewsey at Victoria Park in Warrington and I soon saw why Clock Face had such a bad reputation on the discipline front. You've never seen anything like it. There was a little niggling going on in a tackle and, bingo, one of their players threw a punch. I've never seen thirteen lads dive on someone so quickly in my life. All the Clock Face lads piled in, then the other team came running in. It was a full on brawl. Even the parents joined in and started fighting as well.

Then, one of our lads took the flag off the linesman and started hitting their coach over the head with it. There was about 40 people fighting, I was the only one who didn't join in; I just sat on the touchline watching probably the best fight I have ever seen in my life. I thought 'good on you boys, the other team started it and you've got stuck in'. Our lads didn't take a backward step and the match got abandoned.

We got back into the changing room. I told the lads not to even bother showering; we would go back to Clock Face and shower there. I felt this was the best course of action as Bewsey wanted to carry on fighting.

After every match, we would go in 'The Rec' pub for a drink. Moff returned from a trip to London and I told him we had a bunch of hard lads who wouldn't be picked on, and the next time Bewsey played us they wouldn't start any trouble. We got dragged up in front of the disciplinary at Eccles rugby club. A couple of our players got three and four match bans.

AWARDS AND REWARDS

I suggested to Moff that we bring in some incentives to improve discipline. I'd just finished reading a book about Wigan RLFC when they were dominant in rugby league; they had an award for biggest hit (tackle) in the match. I decided to introduce a similar award for our lads. Bloody hell, it became open season. Moff then came up with the idea of taking them to Blackpool if they didn't finish bottom of the league. My response was one of total horror.

'A load of 15-year-olds to Blackpool for the night, are you insane?'

But he was adamant. So I reluctantly agreed.

We went through the season, up in front of the disciplinary

two or three times. It was like I had a block booking up there. 'Next up, Clock Face. Hello Mark.' It's not bias or looking at it through rose-tinted spectacles but a lot of the time, it wasn't our lads fault. Often, trouble was started, but because they never took a backward step, they got an unfair reputation. Other teams with players that age didn't get involved but with this team, you were picking on the wrong lads.

One lad in particular called Mark Heesome got into a lot of trouble at school and with the police. At 15, he was regularly fighting and beating up blokes twice his age. He was a pretty good player though.

Put it this way, you'd rather have him peeing out of your tent than peeing in it. If you were ever in trouble, you'd want him with you. Yet, Mark was also softly spoken and a pleasant lad who always said 'please' and 'thank you'. However, he was your stereotypical Jekyll and Hyde. When he flipped, he flipped. One day he was suspended from school for fighting with a lad who played for Pilkingtons, the glass company.

We played Pilks and this lad was in their starting line up, so I said to Mark before the match that he wasn't to get involved. Mark promised he wouldn't. Within the first minute, this lad high tackled one of our players and got sent off. When you get sent off, you're meant to go straight to the changing rooms, but this lad stayed on the sidelines.

Then, one of our lads got tackled on their side of the pitch and the Pilks lad ran on the pitch and kicked him in the head. Change of plan was needed now. I told Mark to sort it and sort it he did! Mark went over and pasted him. All their team jumped in, the spectators joined in, it was going off like a frog in a sock. The ref had let little niggles go on throughout the match, so it had escalated. This was the result, a total brawl in the car park; bodies were flying over car bonnets. The fight even spilled into the changing rooms where Mark proceeded to give the lad's dad a good hiding as well.

Match abandoned – and another date with the disciplinary.

The next match, the disciplinary board came down to watch us. We were playing Oldham St Anne's and one of their players started a fight. One of our suspended players ran on from the sidelines and smacked him. I was sat there thinking we were really in trouble now.

And, indeed, at the next night for training the letter from the disciplinary was waiting for us.

When they concentrated on playing rugby though, they were a good team. As the season progressed, we started climbing up the table. We went up to Barrow and they put in a complaint about us because our supporters were 'intimidating'. We'd taken a coach load up who were singing but there was no intimidation or fighting. When Barrow came down to us, they'd heard all these stories about Clock Face being a bunch of thugs and they didn't start any trouble. As they didn't start any, there was none. Barrow's coach talked to us in the pub after the game and said he had heard all these horror stories about us, but he felt they couldn't have been treated better.

We were winning regularly and we went into the last match of the season joint second. We were at home. If we won we'd finish second outright, which would be amazing, considering that we'd been bottom of the league the year before. We drew the game after we scored in the dying seconds. The kick to win the game was right out on the touchline and hit the post. It was enough to get promoted though. The lads came up to me and said 'Yessssss, we're going to Blackpool'.

Oh God, I'd forgotten about that.

The lads all wanted to get tattoos on the trip, so I said that anyone who wanted a tattoo would need to bring me a letter from their parents saying it was all right. There was me, Moff and two other blokes called Ste and Mike who were to take at least twenty 15-year-olds, who just happened to be crazy, to Blackpool for a Saturday night. Everybody in Clock Face was saying: 'This is going to be a nightmare, forget the police, the army are going to be involved. There are going to be ambulances everywhere.'

We went into the Clock Hotel; everyone was saying that I must be crazy. I thought to myself that it might not have been the wisest idea, but we had promised the lads and that was that.

They all turned up, some had letters from their parents giving consent for them to get their tattoos. We drove to Blackpool and got into the hotel. I got all the lads together, just them and me. I told them that if there was any hassle that night, we were finished.

They were all telling me that they would behave. I told them that I trusted them to behave because everybody back at Clock Face was expecting the trip to be a disaster. People were sure some of the lads would return home either in ambulances or cop cars. It was my name on the line, so I stopped Mark and pulled him to one side.

I told him that I was putting him in charge and that when I got up the following morning, I did not want to have to visit a hospital or a police station. If I did, I would hold him responsible. He assured me that it would be fine. I told him not to kid the kidder and that I knew what he was like. He promised that even if he were provoked, there was to be no trouble. Throughout, the season he had never given me a reason not to trust him, he had always done what he had been asked to do. But I was still a bit nervous.

We went to a pub near a tattoo parlour so some of the lads could get their tattoos done. A few of them were playing pool with some blokes in there and an argument started. I shouted my lot over, went over to the blokes and asked them what was up. I knew they had been trying to start trouble, thinking they were only dealing with a bunch of kids. I told the blokes that if they started anything, these kids would rip them to bits and probably leave the pub in rubble.

'Don't be fooled just because they are kids,' I said. 'The reason that they are here is because they are nutters,' I added. I didn't let on that they were a rugby team but said that they were from a young offenders unit on a supervised day out.

I went back over to the lads and got them to forget the argument by starting up a singalong. The blokes backed off and the situation was diffused.

We then went to the 'Manchester' pub because there were strippers on. It was April so it wasn't holiday season and the place was pretty empty. I went to the bouncer and told him that I had a bunch of lads who were only sixteen and asked if it was okay if they came in.

He told me that they could, but if there was any trouble they would get a kicking, same as anybody else. Fair enough, I thought.

There were some Sunday Sport girls in there getting their kit off and the lads were too preoccupied with that to start any trouble. They sat at the front, open-mouthed and dribbling.

We went back to the hotel to get changed and then everyone went out in their own little groups. I re-iterated that I didn't want any trouble. As it happened, I had a great night. I got back to the hotel and heard a bit of shouting and singing later on, but nothing major.

Blackpool had survived. The tower was still standing.

I got up the next morning and every single one of them was down there for breakfast. I didn't mention anything, I just said 'nice one lads'. When we got back to Clock Face, no one could believe that all the lads had come back in one piece with no cuts, bruises or police escorts.

A couple of weeks later, I was talking to one of the lads who played for the team and told him how chuffed I was that there had been no trouble in Blackpool. He told me I had Mark to thank for that. I asked him why and he said that when the lads were coming back from a nightclub they went past a minibus full of Scousers. The Scousers got off and provoked the lads, looking for a fight. Generally, Mark would have been over there like a shot. However, he told the rest of the lads to carry on walking. They were all asking Mark why they hadn't just laid into the Scousers.

'I promised Eccy,' was all he said.

That really meant a lot to me. The incident, as the police would have called it, took place at about 2.30 a.m. Mark was full of ale. Yet he didn't get involved because he had promised me that there would be no trouble. I'll never, ever forget that.

Mark might as well put it in his own words.

Mark Heesome

Mark was absolutely amazing as a coach, when he told you something he would more or less always be right. He knew how to fire us up but also knew when to use his head and calm us down. He knew our faults and would talk us through them.

He put a lot of trust in me because, at the time, I was a Jack the lad but he also saw that I was a decent person. The majority of the lads would always listen to him but I listened to everything properly because I realized he was a wise man. Basically I respected him so much. I think he saw that in me and also knew that he could come to me and ask me to keep an eye on the rest of the lads.

There were times like the trip to Blackpool. Mark said that he would get into a lot of trouble if there were any problems and I should keep an eye on the lads and keep things in order. That's what I did.

Even though I was young at the time of the Blackpool trip in a lot of ways, I had quite an old head on young shoulders and thought 'Jesus Christ, if anything happens on this trip, Mark and Moff are for it'. After Eccy had taken me to one side, it was on my mind that I had to ensure there was no bother.

There was a minibus of Scousers who did try to start trouble with us. What they were saying was fighting talk and normally I would have been the first one in there. They were in their late thirties and one of them in particular was a horrible man. We were getting wound up but I said to the lads, 'Remember what Eccy said and respect his wishes, I know it's hard but walk away.'

If I hadn't have walked away that night, I would have ended up in jail or beaten up. I didn't want anyone to get hurt and I didn't want to let Eccy down. To walk away made me feel like the better person and that I had won the fight without even throwing a punch.

My mum and dad also remember Blackpool.

Pat

Mark didn't tell us what went on at Blackpool. He says to me that if I knew half of what he got up to I'd drop dead. We'll probably only find out a lot of things about what he's got up to from reading the book. Me and Mark have always argued because he's the only one who answers me back!

Jimmy

I used to go down watching him coach Clock Face; he got on well with all the lads too, and he did well with them as well.

PLAYER OF THE YEAR

Not long after Blackpool, we had the Player of the Year awards where we added our own touch with awards such as 'ugliest player of the year' and 'virgin of the year'. Virgin of the year went to one lad who was constantly talking about sex but was still a virgin. We got him a blow up sheep and, in front of all the parents, we made him pretend to make sweet love to it on the dance floor.

I made a speech saying that it had been a fantastic year and that all the doubters out there who had thought Blackpool was going to be a nightmare could now eat their words. I don't think that went down too well with some parents because the event was filmed and that bit was cut out of the video.

The second year we got a couple of better players coming in. One of them should have made it professionally but he discovered that his penis wasn't for stirring tea with. At times when we were ready to go to a match, we would have to track certain players down and drag them out of bed. It was a nightmare sometimes. They'd gone from being 15-year-old kids to 16 and 17-year-old men who had just discovered women and booze.

They were in an under-18s competition so were a little young and received a couple of hammerings. One week, we played Oldham St Annes and brought a ringer in by the name of Gareth Haggerty who would later turn professional. He was on Saints books at the time. I think he scored 6 tries by half time. People were more than inquisitive as to how we had got Haggi to play for us. I just pretended I didn't know what they were talking about, that was quite funny because we got away with it.

The year after when they were 17 and 18, we saw them develop into a very good team. The second season had given them valuable experience. However, the attractions of nightclubs and booze were calling them and it got to the point where we would only have five or six lads turning up for training. I told them that if it didn't pick up, they could forget it because by this time I was full on training for my tennis. I said I wouldn't be rushing back if the turn out continued to be poor. Unfortunately, the situation didn't improve and, in February, we had to wrap the side up.

Looking back though, we had some laughs doing the coaching. I remember the Rec club every Sunday having a drink, taking the lads up to Barrow and them trashing the coach on the way back so much so that the coach firm phoned up the next day to label them 'animals'.

There was one centre called Adam who said he didn't know how to pass the ball so I took him out in the field and showed him how to pass. He went from scoring about 15 tries a season but his winger getting none to his winger getting 15 tries and Adam getting plenty as well. Great player and a hard lad. He had SAS written all over him. You could picture him storming some embassy, shooting five people dead and coming out chewing on a cigar, grinning like a Cheshire cat. He went into the Paratroopers. Tragedy struck Adam though, as he did a parachute jump that went wrong and broke his neck. He's still on his feet but he got discharged from the job he loved. I've had a good chat with him since and he told me that those times at Clock Face were the best of his life.

Adam Langley

Mark was actually one of my references when I joined the Army. The first letter he wrote for me, though, was calling me all sorts! It was a wind up but he soon gave me the real letter. He got me with that one. He has always been an inspiration. I could praise him all day.

TREMENDOUS TIMES AND RICO

I loved training them and I loved Sunday match days. Getting up, picking Moff up for a McDonalds breakfast, watching the match, then going to The Rec for a few jars. Tremendous times.

I remember games away from home where the pitches would be miles away and you would have to go over streams and so on. It was like something out of Cleopatra, as you would have two lads at the front and two lads at the back carrying me shoulder high. The other team wouldn't know what the hell was going on.

They were just misunderstood lads. If someone punched them, they would punch back, fair enough in my book.

Most of them now have turned out to be cracking lads.

The open age team then asked Moff and me if we would coach them because they were having a few problems. We agreed to this, but Moff had lost interest by this point so I was virtually doing it on my own. They were a half decent team. I had been a bit worried that I wouldn't get the respect off the adults that I had got off the kids, but it was fine.

It all ended badly though. In 2001 I went to the Australian Open for the tennis and when I got back, I was told the coaching position was to be advertised in the summer because they wanted a 'high profile name'. I stopped coaching there immediately. There were a couple of people who I feel stabbed me in the back. It's sad because I did a lot for the club. I got them to move the pitch down so they could have a training pitch at the back and got someone to put lights up so they could train in winter. I came up with a few ideas for the clubhouse such as making the changing rooms bigger, which they did. Even now, I think my legacy is still there because a lot of the stuff they've done is stuff that I suggested. A couple of players left because they were upset by how I had been treated.

And to those who did shaft me, I have not forgotten!

I still see quite a few of the lads out and about – they're all grown adults now, some with families. I have great affection for them; I think they feel the same way about me. They always come over, get the beer in and have a chat. The man who was a coach is now a mate.

Before describing my tennis career, I want to mention a friend, David Richards or 'Rico'. We were really good mates and he came to the hospital every week to see me and when I eventually went home, he was always there. We gradually grew apart and fell out over something stupid. I really do regret it now because he, his mum and his dad were really, really good to me. Their friendship and support over the years is something I will never forget and if at any time in the future they need me, I will be there for them. Rico did later ask me to be the best man at his wedding but it was during the qualifying period for Athens 2004 and I was in America. I hope he didn't think I was being funny because I would have done it if I weren't away. I feel really guilty about not being able to do it.

Chapter 10

First Serve

Becoming a tennis player wasn't totally sudden.

When I was playing for Great Britain in the 1993 Wheelchair Rugby International championships at Stoke Mandeville a group of Americans including Rick Draney, Steve Everett and Kevin Whalen put on a wheelchair tennis exhibition. Martin McElhatton from the British Wheelchair Sports Foundation phoned me up and asked me if I would take part in the tennis event.

Wheelchair tennis was founded in 1976. Whilst in rehabilitation an American named Brad Parks came across an article about Jeff Minnenbraker, an athlete from Los Angeles, who had been playing tennis in a wheelchair.

In May 1976, Brad experimented with playing tennis from his wheelchair. Shortly after this, during a routine check-up at hospital, he found that the new recreation therapist was Jeff Minnenbraker. The two started discussing wheelchair tennis. During the spring of 1977 they began to promote the sport across the west coast of the USA.

In May 1977, the Los Angeles City Parks and Recreation Department hosted the first ever wheelchair tennis tournament with around 20 players. Parks and Minnenbraker continued to promote wheelchair tennis through camps, clinics and exhibitions.

By the end of 1980, over 300 players were playing wheelchair tennis in the USA, and potential players in Europe were starting to hear about the sport.

An international team competition, the World Team Cup, was established in 1985, with six men's teams competing. It was played in a similar format to the able-bodied Davis Cup and held on the weekend before the US Open.

As a result of promotional work and demonstrations by Brian Locke of Great Britain and John Noakes of the Netherlands, wheelchair tennis was included in the wheelchair games at Stoke Mandeville in 1987.

At their AGM in July 1988, the International Tennis Federation adopted the 'two bounce rule' into the rules of tennis, officially sanctioning the new sport.

On Monday, 10th October 1988, the International Wheelchair Tennis Federation (IWTF) was founded at a meeting during the US Open in California. All these developments would eventually lead the way for wheelchair tennis to be accepted into the Paralympic Games.

Wheelchair tennis was a demonstration event in the 1988 Summer Paralympics in Seoul, and in 1992 in Barcelona, it acquired the status of a full-fledged competition. Wheelchair tennis fits very easily with the able-bodied game since it can be played on any regular tennis court, with no modifications to rackets and balls. Today, there is an international tour and over 120 annual events. The sport is booming. It has the same rules as able-bodied tennis, with the only exception being that two bounces of the ball are allowed There are three catagories: Men's Open, Women's Open and Quad.

In order to be eligible to compete, a player must have a diagnosed permanent mobility related physical disability. This disability must result in a substantial loss of function in one or both lower extremities. To be eligible to compete in the Quad division, a player must meet the criteria for permanent physical disability and also suffer a substantial loss of function in one or both upper extremities.

Due to the nature of my injury, I would compete in the Quad Division.

Back at Stoke Mandeville I told Martin McEllhatton that I couldn't even hold a racket. Despite that, he asked me if he could put my name down and I said I would have to ask the rugby coach. The coach was Chris Davis and he said to me that if it didn't leave me knackered, I could participate. I went up, watched, and then they showed me how to tape the racket to my hand. When I got to the court, one of the Americans, Kevin Whalen, shouted, 'So you're Eccleston, your reputation precedes you.' He said he had heard about me from the rugby team. Then he invited me on court to hit with him.

The organisers had arranged for a local school to help out with ball kids.

So there we are on court and Kevin Whalen shouts out, 'So which one of you kids is gonna come over and shag our balls?'

I couldn't believe what I had just heard.

I said to him, 'Whooooooooa. You can't say that!'

'We need a ball shagger don't we?' was his reply.

I said that I would very much like a ball shagger but what he had just suggested was illegal in our country.

One of the event organisers came over and explained to Kevin what shagging meant in Britain. He was mortified, the look on his face was priceless and he couldn't apologise enough.

In some parts of the USA, anyone who picks balls up during a tennis match is called a ball shagger.

Later on in my tennis career I was at a tournament in Florida and a player who I now coach was also at the tournament. We were practicing on different courts when a very attractive, fit looking middle-aged woman came over to my court and asked me if I needed a ball shagger. Knowing exactly what she meant, I said I didn't, but the lad on the next court would love it if she would go over and shag his balls.

So off she went and I just sat there watching, crying with laughter, knowing exactly what was about to happen.

She goes over and says, 'Hi, would you like me to shag your balls?'

You should have seen his face!

She pointed over to me and said, 'The guy on the next court said you need your balls shagging.'

By this time I am in tears. He shouts over in a broad Scouse accent, 'Eccy lar, this bird wants to shag me balls!'

I let the situation carry on for a while before I eventually explained to him exactly she meant.

Anyway, back to Stoke Mandeville. I had never played tennis either before my accident or after. So when I played, I got my arse kicked. However, straight after, Rick Draney came up to me. 'You've got to play this game,' he said.

I knew about Rick Draney because he played rugby for San Diego. If you want to sit down and talk about the greatest tetraplegic athlete of all time – it's Rick Draney, with, I beg to suggest, myself in second place.

Draney has a Paralympic gold medal at rugby and has been World No 1 in tennis. He was a fantastic rugby player, very tough and he would give you the same high quality performance every game. He is also the best quad tennis player of all time.

I'm sorry but if anyone says anything to the contrary then they are talking rubbish!

No way am I going to say I was better than Draney as an all round athlete. For him to come up to me after my first attempt at tennis and say I should play the sport meant a hell of a lot to me. Draney was a quiet bloke who would sit, watch, take it all in – and then say something to you later, but always on a one to one basis.

I went away from that week having really enjoyed the tennis and so I began to attend training at Warrington. In 1995 Cyclone, the company who manufacture my wheelchairs, paid for me to go out to the US Open. Stuart, the MD, came with me to study the wheelchairs on display and get an idea of what he would need to design for me.

Stuart Dunne – *Sponsor and MD of 'Cyclone' wheelchairs*

I used to work for a company called Chevron and we got a good deal for Mark to provide him with a sports wheelchair. He hadn't had compensation for his accident so we were glad to help him out. I then started up my own company and it carried on from there. Mark was the first athlete we sponsored.

As for why he has been so successful, some would call it arrogance;

he calls it confidence. I just think that it's bloody-mindedness that has helped him achieve what he has.

I used to train with Mark at Warrington and we used to go round the racing track. Every time we went training and did the 1500 metres Mark would always get me on the final straight!

There was no chance of me beating him.

Rick Draney

I first saw Mark play tennis at an exhibition. Again, the fact that I saw someone with good athletic ability, determination, and good chair skills made me think that Mark could be a good tennis player as well. Plus, I was happy to see some quads (Mark and a few others attended the exhibition/clinic) show an interest in tennis, when most quads were gravitating towards rugby as their sport of choice.

I encouraged him to take up tennis. I think it's always important to be encouraging. I don't know that I ever had any thought or idea about how much he would or would not actually achieve. I knew he had the potential for success – he chose to work hard and I respect his achievements and successes.

I hadn't heard too much about him as a rugby player, in part because I wasn't into rugby as much as I was into tennis from the standpoint of 'knowing the competition.'

WHAT A RACKET

I went out to the US Open for the experience and to see what was involved in what was, for me, a completely new sport. I entered and was convincingly beaten in the first round. Tennis's big attraction was that I had played team sports all my life, and the idea of one-on-one competition really appealed.

It was a fresh challenge and I have always loved challenges so I had to give this a go.

My problem with tennis initially, though, was that I felt that I wouldn't be able to hold the racket properly because my grip wasn't good enough. However, after being shown how to tape the racket, this was no longer an issue.

Another thing that was evident to me, was that I was sat more or less lower than the top of the net which meant I would have to make the ball work more than someone who stands up. As I had to tape the racket to my hand, I was unable to change grip and had to use the same grip for every shot. That made putting spin onto a ball more difficult. I had to find the one ideal grip to hit a forehand, a backhand and a serve. This took me a while because if you didn't get it right, you had a great forehand and a poor backhand or vice versa. Finding a happy medium was probably the most difficult aspect of the game when I started to play seriously.

In November 1996, I entered a tennis tournament in Nottingham. Rob lived in the city so I thought I'd have a few beers with him and see what transpired.

The first day of the tournament, I was sat in the tennis centre with two female umpires. Rob comes in, sees me with these two women and his eyes light up. He has with him the photos from Atlanta – one is very striking, as this masterpiece shows him with a flag coming out of his arse. As you couldn't see Rob's face on the photo we set the girls a little challenge of trying to guess 'who's arse is it anyway?'

We told these girls about our adventures in Atlanta and, although it was against the rules for players to socialise with officials, we arranged to go out with them that night.

Now I am not going to name names, but that very night one of these umpires was straddled across a certain person's lap in a taxi rank and insisted he was to give her a love bite on her breast!

We all went back to Rob's where the party continued until 5 a.m. – and my first match was four hours later!

Have a guess who was umpiring my match?

Once the New Year celebrations were out of the way it was time to become serious and really get into the tennis. I started training at Wavertree and got a coach there by the name of Craig Jones. That's where it all started off.

Craig moved from Wavertree to Wirral so I moved over with him and he got a really good wheelchair tennis programme going. As with rugby, money was a problem.

I wrote lots of letters to try and get money to fund my tennis career because back then there was no lottery funding available. The British Tennis Foundation weren't interested so I needed sponsors. I won't mention the person's name because it will probably embarrass them but someone who came training with us told me that their brother worked in a bank and the bank gave money to athletes every year. I thought nothing of it. One day, I returned home from training and unzipped my racket bag to find an envelope. There was a card inside saying 'Mark, my brother from the bank has given me this cheque to give you'.

The majority of people who have spinal cord injuries get compensation these days, sometimes to the tune of millions. Back then, I got nothing. I was skint. I think this person realised that I was struggling and that I needed a helping hand. I might be wrong but I have a suspicion that it was a very kind and wonderful human being rather than a bank that actually gave me the money.

Either way, I will never forget what they did for me.

If they ever read this, they will know who I am talking about and I want them to know I am eternally grateful.

Thank You!

That cheque paid for my trip to Japan in May 1998. This was an important tournament because all the players I needed to beat to start getting noticed were there. This could be my break through; this could be the big time. It might make people sit up and take notice.

Getting to Japan was a pain. There was an 8 hour flight to Hong Kong then a 6-hour wait for the flight to Fukuoka where the tournament was being held. Then another 2 hour flight, then a 2 hour drive from the airport to where I was staying. I was knackered by the time I got to the hotel. The saving grace was that the hotel and tennis centre were on the same site. I shared a room with Steve Wood, who at the time was a wheelchair tennis player and my training partner. He was very knowledgeable about tennis.

Steve had tips for me and he ran through the plan of what I should do if I had to play against the World No 1, Brian Hanson.

I battered Hanson in the final 6–4 6–2.

He was gutted and spat the dummy out big time. My big break had happened. When I got back, all of a sudden, everyone was interested in me. Here started my climb up the tennis ranks.

Throughout it, I was motivated as ever. If something was going on at the sidelines, I reacted. I'd confront the situation. People say I had a bit of McEnroe about me in that I took no hostages, but if someone was doing something that affected me, I wanted to know why – and I wanted it sorted out there and then.

Chapter 11

Second Serve

Melinda Messenger, Caprice, Anthea Turner, Zoe Ball, Kelly Brook ... oh and me.

Littlewoods sponsored us all.

When I realised I wanted to get seriously involved in tennis, I sent out hundreds of letters asking for sponsorship. I was getting the odd £25 cheque but that was about it. Then I received a letter from Littlewoods saying they were really interested in what I had to say and would I come in and talk to them.

I went to Littlewoods in Liverpool and explained that I had been captain of the Great Britain wheelchair rugby team, that I had switched to tennis and just won the Japan Open. I told them my aim was to climb the rankings and become World No 1. They said that if my letter had landed on their doorstep any other day it would have been binned. But it arrived at the time they were getting a new Chief Executive who wanted to boost the home shopping market. They told me they were interested. The conversation went as follows:

Littlewoods: *'How does twelve suit you?'*

Me: *'Twelve hundred would be great, thanks.'*

Littlewoods: *'Not twelve hundred, twelve thousand.'*

I pretended not to be shocked. I scratched my chin as if I was considering whether it was an acceptable offer.

Littlewoods: *'Does twelve grand cover it, Mark?'*

Me: *'Er... Yes that's great... Thank you.'*

Cover it? I felt like shouting back to them that I had just wet myself. I couldn't believe it. But I accepted the offer in a very cool and calm manner. All the while I was cart-wheeling in my mind. I could not believe what I had just heard.

It was at this time I first met Lucy. We went out for a while, then she dumped me. Dump me? How dare she! To be fair though we did both have other things going on, so it was probably a good move.

We met up again a couple of years later. She is probably the most honest and caring person I have ever met, way too nice for me!

Littlewoods told me that the offer did have one condition. The condition was that I go down to London, all expenses paid, to do a photo shoot for the Littlewoods catalogue.

Oh go on then, if I must!

I had to become a male model.

I was put up in a posh London hotel the night before I did the photo shoot with Derek Redmond, the ex 400 metre runner. I had to do all the daft catalogue poses. This got me some serious stick from my mates, but for twelve grand I couldn't give a monkey's.

My mates blew some of the photos up and put them up in the Clock Hotel. The deal funded all my tournament travel and enabled me to buy a load of new equipment.

The second year of the contract was torture. I had to go on a photo shoot with Kelly Brook. Tough job but someone had to do it. They also upped my money to £15,000. I had to travel to London for the catalogue launch again. They picked me up from my house in a chauffeur driven Lexus and drove me all the way to a yet another posh hotel in London where I stayed. I had to have a slap up dinner with all the top executives; I felt like a film star – it was amazing.

The next day was the catalogue launch at a 'we don't let you in if you look like a scruff' wine bar opposite St James's Palace. I was on a table with Alan Hanson, Kelly Brook and the Littlewoods' hierarchy. All I had to do was to sit there in Adidas gear and smile.

As I say, tough, tough work. But, somehow, I got through it.

They gave me an agent to sort out all the press releases. Two year deal – £27,000, get in there!

This was before lottery funding so it paid for everything and, in sport, money does matter. Littlewoods' funding enabled me to climb the rankings rapidly.

The tennis scene was changing, as there was a lot of pressure to include Quad tennis in major competitions. It finally happened in Barcelona 1998 when the quad division was included in the World Team Cup for the first time. The World Team Cup is the Davis Cup of wheelchair tennis.

Steve Wood rang me with the news that the Quad division was included and I was heading to Barcelona. It was a four-team competition. Great Britain, USA, France and Japan battled it out in a round robin with the top two meeting in the final.

It was amazing. I had done International Games and the Paralympics with the rugby but I had never experienced anything like this. The way it was organised was so professional. It was one of the most enjoyable tournaments I have ever been involved in. One reason was that I was treated like a professional athlete.

The centre was tremendous. We were given a driver who stayed with us during our time there. We christened him 'Loco' as he was absolutely nuts. He was only about 23 – and hilarious and wanted to be in Formula 1.

He would drive round bends at about 90 miles per hour. He took us to nightclubs and taught us what we thought were Spanish chat up lines. In fact, they were really very rude comments that resulted in me getting slapped once.

We played France and Japan and beat them both. Then we played America in the group stage. I had gotten to know the American players pretty well along with their coach, Jason Harnett. Jason is one of the most genuine blokes you could ever wish to meet, a legend as far as I'm concerned.

I played Draney. I had never beaten him in God knows how many attempts. But my luck seemed to be changing. I won the first set 6–1. Everyone was gob-smacked because Draney was No 1 in the world. I lost the second set though.

The third set started tentatively as both of us didn't want to make any errors and give any edge to the other. However, this soon changed and we both resorted to the type of battle that we had had in the previous two sets. To be honest, I felt confident at this point but when you're playing such a great player as Draney, it is always in the back of your mind that there is a reason he is the best in the world.

The set went with serve. So the match was to be decided by a tiebreak. A lot of people say that a tiebreak is a lottery but I think those that do don't like playing them, never practice them or are talking rubbish.

I went into the tiebreak knowing that the winner would be the one who made the least number of errors. Neither of us made many mistakes. At 6–5 I had a match point against him but, as I've already mentioned, there was a reason that Draney was number one. He was one of those players who could turn a match in the blink of an eye. At this point I began to think too much of the enormity of the situation I was in.

MATCH POINT AGAINST DRANEY!

As a result I tightened up, made the error and ended up losing but I came off the court very happy that I had put in such a strong performance. I was relatively new to the sport and I had just taken the greatest Quad player ever all the way to the wire. We had held nothing back against each other and it was an absolute honour to be involved in probably the best tennis match I've ever played in. Even though I lost, I realised in those two to three hours I had earned the right to mix it with the world's best.

Jason Harnett has coached players who have played at Wimbledon, he has coached juniors who have gone on the World tour, he works with a coach who used to work at the Nick Bollettieri academy in Florida, so he is a man who knows a thing or two about tennis. He told me that, at any level anywhere, that that singles match between me and Draney is up there with the best tennis matches he has ever seen.

We played the USA in the final and I played Hanson. It was really hot and I struggled badly with the heat.

NO SWEAT

Most complete injury tetraplegics, are unable to sweat due to the damage to the spinal cord. Because I couldn't sweat my body would overheat very rapidly. The best way to explain it would be to imagine having no water in your car and driving off. After a while your car will overheat and come to a stand still. That's exactly what would happen to me. I have lost a number of matches simply from overheating.

Some people just didn't realise to what extent this affected me. Once, after the final in Sydney in 2002, I had to be given oxygen as I started to see spots, feel sick, slur my words and had absolutely no energy whatsoever. At tournaments I would regularly go back to my hotel room and be so ill I would throw my guts up. I was constantly pouring cold water over my head to keep cool. I think out of all the players on the tour, I probably suffered from the heat most of all.

I even once did a study at Brighton University on how heat affects tetraplegics and the benefits of using ice vests. I had to go into a heat chamber and do a work out for an hour without using an ice vest. Then, I had to go in after having an ice vest on for half an hour before, and then, I did an hour with the vest on. I turned out to be an interesting scientific specimen.

When I did it without using the vest at all, I had to ask to come out after 30 minutes.

When I did it after having the vest on before I went in, I had to ask to come out after 40 minutes.

When I did it with the ice vest on I felt fine but I was taken out after 50 minutes, as the readings showed that my core temperature was over the legally allowed limit for the trial. With hindsight now I think that in some tournaments my core temperature got so high that I probably was in real danger.

In one match – and I'm proud it has only been one match – I had to give up. That was in a doubles match in Australia in 2001. I was so hot I felt sick and couldn't see properly. We won the first set but I said to my partner that if we lost the second set, I was off.

We lost it – so I quit. I am no quitter but I honestly believe, knowing what I know now, that if I hadn't have stopped then I would have been in serious trouble.

I got that concerned about losing matches due to the heat that I went to speak to Dr Clive Glass who is the Clinical Psychologist at the Spinal Unit in Southport. It was upsetting me that my physical condition, and not my technical ability, was the reason I would occasionally lose to people who, quite frankly, I would normally beat easily.

Dr Clive Glass *agrees*

Mark came to speak to me concerning his inability to deal with high temperatures. After chatting with him I determined that because he was getting so hot and he wanted to get out of there, he was guilty of occasionally rushing his shots. Whilst this was in part due to his temperament it was mainly due to hot climate, where unless he finished games quickly, he would fade and lose.

Back in Barcelona in 1998, the heat was unbelievable. The first set in my match against Hanson went to a tiebreak, which I lost. I couldn't concentrate and just kept thinking that I needed to get out of the sun. I lost the second set 6–0.

I got battered and we lost the final.

Jason Harnett was the only coach who really knew how to beat me and he beat me on a regular basis. I spoke to him after the final and asked him why he had put Hanson in the final against me instead of Draney. He said it was because earlier in the year I had beaten Hanson in the Japan Open final and Hanson wanted revenge – badly. I didn't achieve what I wanted to achieve because, obviously, we had wanted to win the competition. But getting match point against Draney earlier in the tournament was a huge positive for me to take away.

I've worked with lots of coaches over the years and at the very top are Brian Worrall, Terry Vinyard and Jason Harnett. Although Jason never directly coached me, I have hit with him. We're friends and we still keep in touch even though he lives in California. I have a lot of respect for Jason.

He is a class act.

He would never rub it in when he had coached someone to beat me. He'd be the first to give me a hug after a game. You could take that as patronising from some people but not from Jason. Whenever he spoke I listened.

I would have loved to have worked with him. I believe he could have made me an even better player.

Jason Harnett – *US Paralympic Tennis Coach*

I first met Mark at the US Open back in 1997. He was an obstinate fellow. When all the players I knew told me that he was one to watch, I could see that his competitiveness was his strength.

The match between Mark and Rick Draney was the best match I have ever seen, well, maybe the second. I think the 1996 Masters Final between Pete Sampras and Boris Becker may have the edge, but, truly, Mark and Rick's match was as good a match as I have ever witnessed in person and been a part of as a coach. It had all of the classic qualities necessary for greatness.

A great rivalry between two great players played out on the court. This was an enormous moment in the history of Quad tennis, as it was the final of the inaugural World Team Cup in Barcelona.

Mark was a difficult player to coach against. You always knew that he would fight tooth and nail to win. It was a matter of reading his energy levels, his temperament and understanding his disability. There was no question that Mark's heart and desire to succeed overwhelmed any disability he had. He could literally will himself to win in most matches. That is a trait that you cannot teach as a coach. You either have it or you don't. Rick Draney also had those qualities.

That was what made their match in Barcelona so great. I truly believed that Mark hated losing more than he loved winning. He also had one of the best forehands in the game, especially at shoulder height.

I think sometimes his desire to avoid a loss, not the winning part, drove him to be a nasty competitor as well. It was not always directed at the opponent, but sometimes at the officials. I always saw it as his competitive nature coming out, not necessarily as a tactic of taking his opponent out of their game. Though I am sure it did do that at times as a side effect.

I would rate Mark as one of the best ever tennis players of wheelchair tennis. I have always said that the Quads produce great tennis players. Because they cannot hit the ball as hard as the Paraplegic division players do, I believe it has forced them to become true students of the game and to play this sport with a level of intelligence only shown by the best of the Para division. Even though Mark did not win multiple titles of the big tournaments (US Open, Japan Open, British Open . . .), he was one of a handful of players who I would consider truly excellent tennis players, not just players who play tennis.

My list includes in the men's game: Randy Snow, David Hall, Rick Draney, Brian Hanson, David Wagner, Nick Taylor, Robin Ammerlaan.

And in the women's, Esther Vergeer and Daniela di Toro

Mark loved the competition and always rose to the occasion.

Our relationship was more on a professional level than social. We both wished we could have hung out more, but at these events, our obligations were to our teams. If we shared a meal together we would always 'have a laugh', but most of our experiences together were on the court. His humour though always made me laugh.

If I were to describe Mark to someone who didn't know him, I would tell them about his competitiveness and his desire to win. Mark has always been a nice man (off the court!) and always retained his humour. He was fiercely loyal to those close to him and I suspect it is no different at home with his friends and family. He is a player I will miss not having around at the tournaments, because I feel we had a mutual respect and understanding for one another that is not only hard to find in sport, but in life as well.

My opponent has memories of that epic too and has been kind enough to share them with me.

Rick Draney *recalls*

The game against Mark in Barcelona was more than a classic moment, and it was more than a classic match against Mark. For the first time, quads were being included at the World Team Cup. I had been lobbying and politicking since the early 90s for us to be internationally recognized as a division and included at international competitions. Finally, we were legitimized in tennis as athletes. This was a significant milestone and, thankfully, the beginning of things to come internationally for quad tennis players. I think every quad tennis player there in Barcelona recognized the significance of the moment and was intent on 'putting on a good show', and proving that we were deserving of the opportunity and inclusion. This was our first chance in tennis to represent our countries and the only chance to be the first quad champions at the World Team Cup. For these reasons, and due to the competitive desire both Mark and I possessed, each of us really, really, really wanted to win!

It wasn't necessarily the greatest match ever just in terms of the tennis being played. I thought we both played very well (I managed to play a little better) and there were a lot of good shots and good points. But, it goes back to the significance of the moment. It brought out a higher level of determination and passion, a greater sense of tension and urgency. The combination of the tennis and the drama associated with essentially, the beginning of the history of quad tennis internationally made it such a memorable match.

Early on in our matches, I had the edge in experience and confidence, so I did not feel pushed or threatened by Mark. I recognized his passion for the game and knew that if he kept after it, it would only be a matter of time before he would start to pose a 'problem' for me and other top players. Sure enough, he indeed became a 'problem' for me and other top players, as he became a top player himself. He was no longer just a problem – he was a legitimate threat (and a bit of a nuisance).

CLASS ACT

I always got on well with Draney. He was a class act too. He lost with grace and wouldn't come up with excuses. He had to pack the tennis in due to a problem with his wrist. The whole Quad division and, indeed, anyone who plays wheelchair tennis owes Rick Draney a great debt, because he championed the division and pushed for it to be included in the World Team Cup, and then in the Paralympics. I consider it an injustice that he didn't get to play in Athens because it was the first Paralympics our division was involved with.

Draney had suffered a wrist injury, which affected his form to the extent that he didn't meet the US qualification criteria for Athens, but he should have been given a wildcard entry. I sent him an e-mail saying it felt strange, being there without him. If it wasn't for him doing exhibitions, demonstrations and attending numerous meetings we would never have been included at Athens. The first time I beat him was in Holland in 2000 after God knows how many attempts. He congratulated me very warmly and said some really kind words.

The man is a gentleman.

Hanson was a different animal, a strange puppy. He never got on with many people. Draney and Hanson hated each other's guts. I think Hanson, when he was No 1, got on the cover of Sports Illustrated and Draney resented that, or was it the other way round? Not sure, but they never spoke.

Hanson was a PE teacher and liked soccer, so he would chew my ear off about my beloved Liverpool. I was one of the few on tour who got on with him. I seem to be one of these people who gets on with people who are described as strange by others. Maybe it's because I'm a weirdo! Although I prefer to think I'm a good judge of character.

However, in Barcelona, when he beat me in the final, Hanson came rushing up to the net giving it all this 'yeah, baby, in your face'. I was taken aback and not at all impressed.

It was really out of order, especially as he knew I was struggling with the heat. Even Jason said it was out of order and a couple of the Americans, including Draney, would later say they were embarrassed by it and apologized. I fell out with Hanson over this and I let him know my feelings when I went past him. I simply told him I had thought better of him and that he had no class.

Hanson had a bit of a chip on his shoulder and gave the impression that he felt the world was against him. He had been a very good lacrosse player before his accident and, maybe, he was a little bitter. I don't know. It was a shame he did what he did because I used to enjoy talking to him.

The next time I played him was at the US indoor final in Milwaukee and I started doing the whole 'in your face' routine to him. The crowd had been giving it the USA chant. So when I won, I looked over at them and said 'in your face'.

Looking back, I'm lucky they didn't lynch me on the spot.

Steve Everett, another US tennis player, was close to Hanson and told me that he really regretted what had happened in Barcelona. I told Steve that if Hanson apologised it would all be forgotten. The apology never came, despite many opportunities. It was a shame really because he didn't have many friends on the circuit, so what he did in Barcelona didn't make any sense to me.

Chapter 12

So Near and Yet So Far

In April 1999 I entered the Florida Open, knowing that if I won I had a great chance of becoming World No 1.

I was world No 3 by this point. Hanson and Draney were No 1 and No 2 respectively, but Draney hadn't turned up for the tournament.

I knew I had a bit of an 'Indian sign' over Hanson as I had beaten him more often than not. So the opportunity to take top spot was there. But when I arrived in Florida I felt very weak and strange. I did a quick practice session, returned to the hotel to change and then went to the shopping mall.

The hotel shuttle bus took us to the mall but the bus was quite high and I had to lift myself into it. It was at this point that my problems began. As I was pushing myself round the shopping mall, my right arm was getting weaker and weaker. At first I put it down to the travelling.

I got back to my hotel room and realised this was more than jet lag or fatigue; something was very wrong. I showed my roommate my arm and said I had trouble moving my hand. The next morning I couldn't move my right hand at all.

My immediate fear was that it was syringomyelia (or syrinx). A syrinx is a fluid-filled cavity that develops in the spinal cord, in the brain stem, when it is called a syringobulbia, or in both.

Syrinxes that grow in the spinal cord press on it from within. Although most common in the neck, a syrinx can occur anywhere along the length of the spinal cord and often extends to affect a long segment of the cord. Usually, the nerves that detect pain and temperature changes are most affected. Cuts and burns are common, because people with this type of nerve damage cannot feel pain or heat. As a syrinx extends further, it can cause spasms and weakness, usually beginning in the arms. Eventually, the muscles supplied by the affected nerves may begin to waste away.

I was convinced this was what I had. If I was right, it would require surgery fast, in which a shunt is placed in your neck and the fluid is drained.

I went to see the tournament nurse and told her I also had a sharp pain in my back. She sent me to see the doctor who arranged for me to have an MRI scan that day.

I was driven to a university and was placed on the scanner. To be frank, I was shitting myself because I really thought it was a syrinx and that petrified me.

I got my results immediately. The doctor told me I had a syrinx.

My worst nightmare had come true.

I was terrified. I rang the spinal unit back home and explained what had happened. My doctor, told me to get the first flight home. The doctor in the US told me that if I wanted the operation there he would arrange it.

Er, thanks but no thanks.

I just wanted to get home as fast as possible.

Waiting when you are petrified is awful. I couldn't get a flight for two days. It was horrible. God bless Simmo who shared a room with me, he helped me with everything, including packing and getting dressed. He even brought me a cup of tea, while I was sat on the toilet listening to Keith Sweat.

But if Simmo was great, then the organisers were bang out of order. They charged me $50 for the ride to the airport and I had to lug all my kit myself, which is very difficult when you can't move your right arm properly. I had to get my tennis chair, my racket bag and my holdall over to check-in myself. It was a nightmare.

I don't really remember much about the flight home. I just went into autopilot. I flew from Miami to Heathrow, scuttled to Terminal 1 and flew to Manchester.

I went straight to the Spinal Unit and showed them my MRI scans. As they had MRI scans for me from a couple of years before, they were able to see the damage.

My consultant, Mr Soni compared both sets of scans and gave me the first hope. He thought that it was possible that the training, the playing, the wear and tear of working out, might have caused some neurological damage. He couldn't see much difference in the two scans so he wasn't convinced it was a syrinx. More likely, he thought, it was a disc problem.

Eventually Mr Soni concluded that the problem was caused by a disc protrusion at C5/C6 level, which contributed to a pincer effect on the spinal cord. The fusion at C6/C7 level of my vertebrae and overcompensating disc damage at C5/C6 level (with the protrusion) was the likely cause of the neurological loss. You have got no idea how relieved I was to find out that it wasn't what the American doctor had said it was.

I was in hospital for two weeks and they put me on intravenous anti-inflammatory steroids.

I received some special visitors whilst in hospital, a group of testosterone loaded 19-year-old lads who had played rugby for me at Clock Face! The hospital didn't know what hit them. Every nurse that walked past got a chorus of raucous comments from the lads. It was hilarious.

But the truth was bleak. I had lost quite a bit of the use of my right hand permanently.

Mr Soni told me to go home and not do anything for six weeks and then go back and see him. I completely lost the plot. I thought my tennis career was over since I couldn't move my right hand much. All this when I was so close to becoming world No 1.

When I went home, I felt weak all of the time and couldn't do much for six weeks. I just lay on the bed watching telly day and night. Believe me if you have to lie around and watch hours of soap, dope and mope telly, you become very motivated to get off that bed and stop being a potato. I decided that I had come so close to achieving my goal there was no way I was packing it in. I was carrying on. I told Mr Soni and he told me to achieve what I wanted to achieve – and then call it a day. He knew it was what I wanted and he supported my decision 100%.

But the injury meant I had to change my style of play as I had lost movement and strength in my right hand. That loss of movement and power meant I was no longer able to hold the ball the way I used to when I was serving. So, for the first few weeks my ball toss was all over the place. Also, I couldn't grab the push rim on my right wheel like I did before and had to push with my right hand nearly clenched. It took a while for me to adjust to these new physical obstacles.

Foolishly I was too keen to get back. I played the British Open in July, which with hindsight, I should never have done. I was nowhere near ready.

I wrote to Littlewoods explaining my situation and offered to pay my money back but they refused, said that I could keep it and wished me luck. When I came back to playing, I wrote to them once more but all the people I had been dealing with had left the company and I never heard from them again.

World Team Cup was coming up in August at Flushing Meadow, New York and I was asked if I would be ready to play there. I knew I wouldn't be. I was gutted to miss the opportunity to play at such a magnificent venue.

I had a couple of months off and then did the Nottingham tournament at the beginning of November. I was playing in the semi final and I won the first set and was 5–0 up in the second set. Then total disaster. My arm became weak and my hand started to go into spasm. Not surprisingly, I lost the match. The result was dramatic. You had all the idiots running round saying that I had choked. Even one of the Great Britain coaches, someone who is the worst coach I have ever had the misfortune of meeting, said I had choked. Now he may have been joking when he said this but it was not very tactful or subtle and he said it in front of other players, not the kind of thing I expected from a national coach. Brian Worral certainly would not have been so insensitive.

I had some more time off after this and got myself together. This time I became more patient, realising that if I rushed back again the consequences could be even more devastating. I rested, trained sensibly and took my time; something that I should have done initially.

By 2000 I was well enough to start playing again and I began to climb up the rankings. In April I went to Japan and won the tournament. This made my intentions pretty clear – I was back and if any idiot thought I was a choker they would soon find out on court. I got to 7th on the world rankings.

In 2001, I went back to Florida. I got to the final and played Studwell, another American and a left-hander. The Great Britain Quad coach had to go home before the final so we had arranged for another Great Britain coach (the one who called me a choker) to warm me up for the final. I was due to meet him for breakfast at 7 a.m.

He told me if he were not there at 7 a.m, he would meet me, ready to go, at the tennis centre at 8 a.m. The final was at 9 a.m.

At 7 a.m. I started having breakfast, no sign of him.

At 8 a.m I got the transport across to the tennis centre, and, you guessed, there was still no sign of him.

I got strapped up and I was sat on court waiting for him, no sign of him. He never turned up, in fact.

At ten to nine I had to un-strap to go to the toilet and get ready for the final at 9 o'clock. I was livid. Here I am in the final of a major tournament and there is no sign of the Great Britain coach who is supposed to be warming me up. I went out on court absolutely furious, not the ideal emotion to feel as you're about to play in a final.

I played the final and lost. I am not one for making excuses but I don't think what happened before the game put me in the best frame of mind for competing. Coach eventually blessed us with his presence at about 1 p.m. and had a big, pathetic, clownish grin on his face.

He told me he was sorry.

I told him to fuck off.

He said he could understand I was upset but his alarm hadn't gone off.

Later that day, I was talking to another player, someone who I have no reason whatsoever to doubt; he told me that he had been in a club the night before and surprise, surprise, guess who he said was in there with him. Yep, our very own Mr Alarm Clock with No Ringing Tone. The one who had the nerve to call me a choker.

I wonder if he has ever won anything.

I was even more livid after this.

I have partied plenty before events but I pride myself on always being professional and always showing up – ready for action whether it be rugby or tennis.

When I got home, I was on the phone immediately to Sue Wolstenholme, the head of the British Tennis Foundation. She said she had spoken to the coach and, although it was unfortunate, these things did happen so that was the end of the matter. I brought up a conversation I had with someone who claimed the Coach was in a club, only to be told that we were not going to start discussing rumours and speculation. It was totally swept under the carpet. I did not even get an apology. If it had been the other way around, I would have been kicked off the program and never played again.

Then, we got to the World Team Cup in Switzerland in September 2001 and, again, I saw behaviour that I felt just wasn't right. Behaviour that upset a very good friend of mine, and if you upset a friend of mine then you upset me.

Some coaches in wheelchair tennis that I have come across just don't have a clue.

Switzerland in September 2001 was the first World Team Cup that Pete Norfolk was involved in. He is a paraplegic but he had a syrinx, which caused him to lose some function in his right hand. This was also the first world team cup to be coached by James Pankhurst.

In May 2001, I had gone to Japan and won. I then went straight to play in three tournaments in the USA. Alabama, St Louis and Atlanta. The announcement of Pankhurst getting the job was made while I was in Japan; I suspect they wanted me out of the way as my coach Craig Jones had also applied for the job. I knew they didn't like him and so I knew that he was not going to get the job. I also made it clear that I wouldn't be happy with

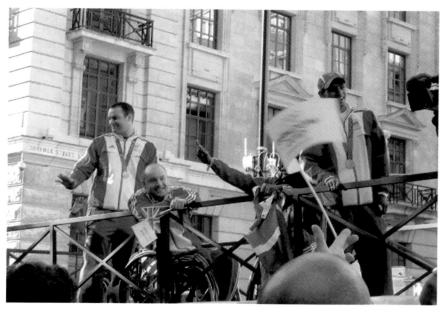

Parade of Champions.

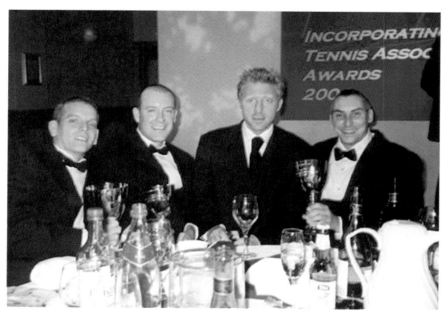

ITA Team of the Year.

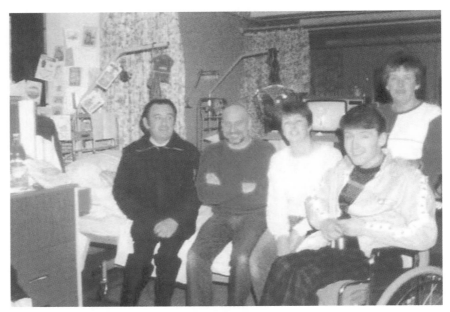

Just after the accident.

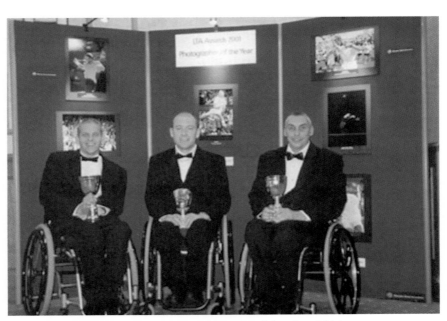

World Team Cup winners celebration 2001.

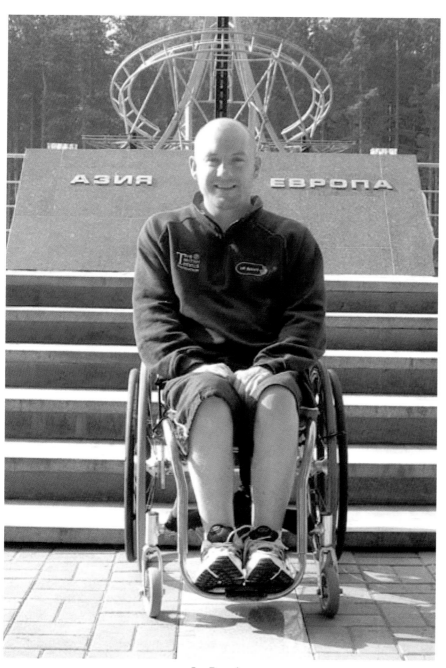

In Russia.

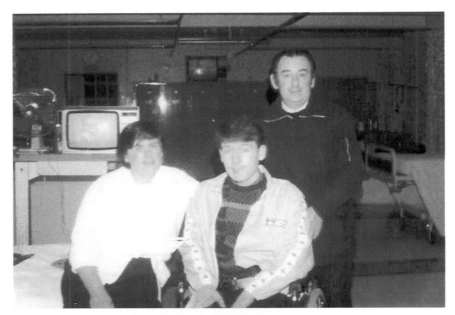

With mum and dad in hospital.

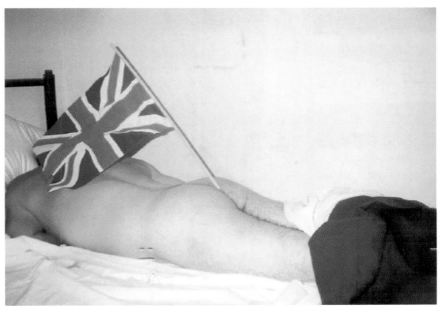

At the Atlanta Paralympics, patriotic Rob Tarr.

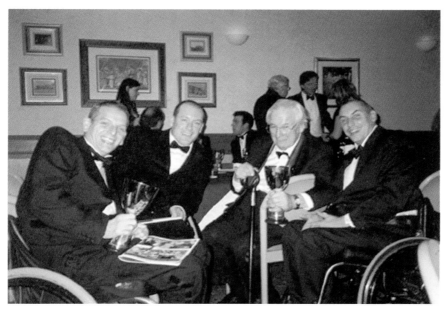

With Sir Peter Ustinov, the great entertainer.

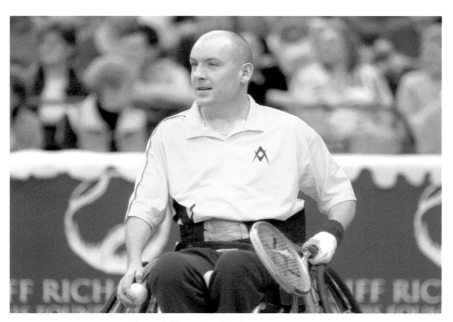

At the Cliff Richard Classic Tournament.

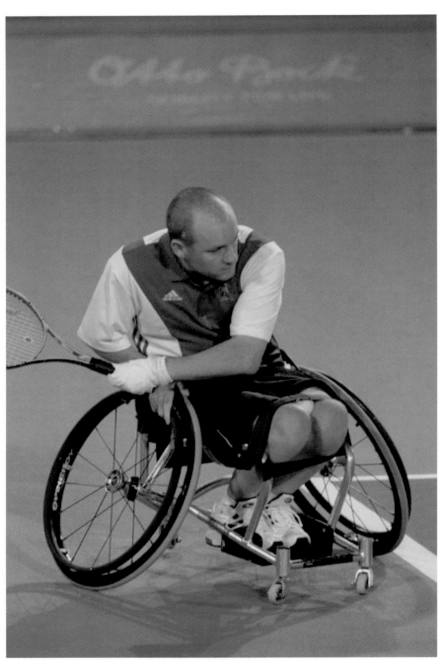

Who says I don't have a good backhand?

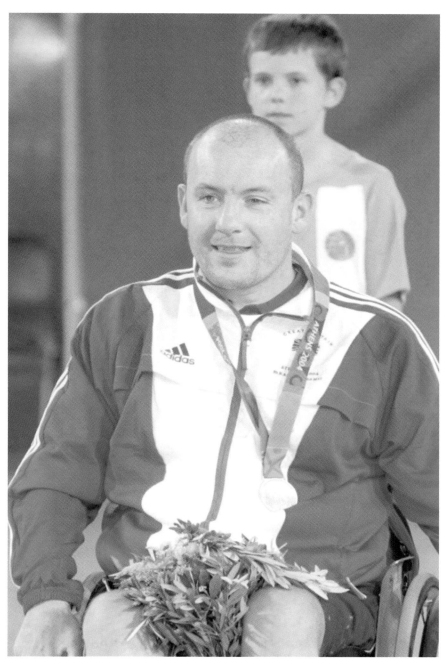

Me and my medal.

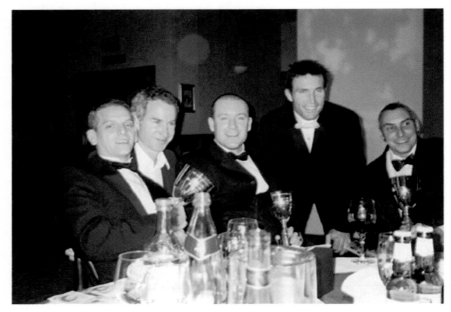

With John McEnroe and Pat Cash.

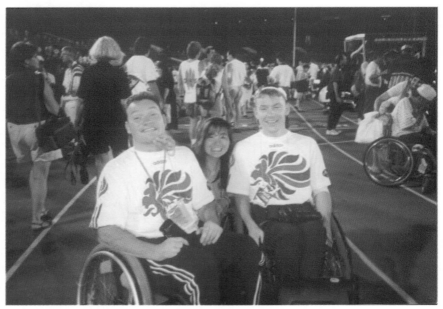

At the Atlanta Paralympics, Rob and Mark's excellent adventure.

the appointment of a man I felt did not know enough about wheelchair tennis. However, he proved to be a good coach and will eventually go on to become a great coach.

At the time though I felt he was given the job too early in the respect that he had to deal with two huge egotistical maniacs like Pete Norfolk and me.

In Switzerland, Israel were favourites; they were very strong and had won it the year before. They were nasty as well.

There were two groups of four. We were in a group with Canada, Holland and Israel. That week, I played the best tennis of my life. I cleaned out everybody I met. The rules are simple. Each country has a No 1 player and a No 2 player.

Your No 2 will play your opponent's No 2 first, then the No 1's play each other. If the score is one-all, you then play a doubles decider.

I was Britain's No 1 player. We played Canada first. Pete Norfolk beat his opponent pretty easily. I played Hunter, a top five player at the time and won comfortably.

We played Holland and Pete Norfolk won pretty easily, I played Bas Van Erp, a top five player, who had beaten me easily the week before in Geneva. This time I cleaned him out.

I hammered both my opponents.

We then played Israel. The winner would go through to the final. In the other group USA were up against Japan. We expected America to progress. Pete won his match against Haim Lev, who I did not like one bit. I was next up against Weinberg and any time I went to hit a shot, Lev would shout out something in Hebrew. He was also crunching a water bottle during my serve. I looked at the Umpire wondering why he was not doing anything about this. The Israelis pushed it, simple as that. Whenever they were losing a match they would cause all kinds of grief or fake an injury to disrupt your momentum. Lev was a master of these tactics. I turned round and smacked the ball straight at him. Unfortunately it hit the net curtain that he was sat behind. He gave me the evil eye. He carried on crunching the water bottle.

One of the women players on our team used to be a nurse in Saudi Arabia and she went over and said something to Lev in

Arabic. He spat on the floor in front of her and began to express his undoubted hatred of anything Arab. Pete went and sat next to him, grabbed the water bottle off him and threw it on the floor. So now, Lev had Pete sat one side of him and the nurse on the other. He soon shut up.

I lost the first set, 6–3. At the end of the first set, Dawn Newbury, the Great Britain team manager, was sat just behind James Pankhurst and she looked worried.

Now let me say right here that I know more about open-heart surgery than a lot of wheelchair tennis coaches know about wheelchair tennis. For example, there was one Great Britain coach who told me that when I played Draney I should go to his forehand. Rick Draney had the best forehand in world tennis. Hitting a ball to his forehand is like telling Man United opponents to keep giving the ball to Wayne Rooney or Ronaldo.

Anyway, Pankhurst was trying to encourage me. I think he was getting concerned but I wasn't worried at all. A lot of people panic if they go a set down but my thinking is if you lose the first set, so what? You have to win two sets to win a match, so your situation hasn't changed.

I told James not to worry, as I knew once I got my returns in, the match would be over and Britain would be in the final. Anyway I found my returns and I won.

Against the formbook, Japan had beaten America in the semis so they would be our opponents. Tachibana was one of their top players but he had only ever really got as far as quarter-finals of tournaments before. Now people were starting to see him as a potential major force in the sport.

I played him and was on fire in the first set winning it 6–1. However, I was 5–2 down in the second set, but pulled it back to 6–6 and we had to play a tiebreak, which I won.

We had won the World Team Cup, the first British team to do so.

Although the World Team Cup is a team event and Pete Norfolk was part of that first Great Britain team to win the world team cup, my performances were the major reason we triumphed.

At the Lawn Tennis Association awards in 2001, they had a

disabled player of the year award, which they gave to us as a team after we had won the cup for the first time. We went down to Wimbledon to get the award. Boris Becker, Pat Cash and John McEnroe were all there. They were all all right; they came over, sat with us and had a chat.

They were very complimentary about wheelchair tennis and agreed that the sport deserved a lot more media coverage than it was getting. A challenge to a game in a wheelchair was issued but politely declined.

The following year, we went again to the awards and Peter Ustinov was the speaker. They were great nights and we were treated well. I have been to a number of presentation ceremonies, a couple of which I found slightly patronising, but this wasn't patronising at all; it was a reward for our achievements.

Chapter 13

Game, Set and Match

In November 2001 I decided that I had gone as far as I could with my coach Craig. He had just started a new job and it was getting more and more difficult for him to fit sessions in.

I was a bit worried about telling him because he was also a mate and had been my coach since day one. It turned out he actually agreed with me.

Craig wasn't everybody's cup of tea, especially not the British Tennis Foundation's, but he was a very good tennis coach. He deserves a lot of credit for my achievements because he taught me a hell of a lot, but as eventually happens with every coach/player relationship, we had gone as far as we could.

Success paid dividends. I secured another substantial sponsorship deal with a company called Anixter. This enabled me to get more equipment and play more tournaments.

I started working with my new coach, Phil Leighton. Phil brought a fresh and different approach. He is a PCA coach; it stands for Professional Coaching Award, the highest level tennis coach in the UK.

What a lot of people don't realise is that I only hit with Phil three hours a week. He wouldn't hit with me any more that that.

When I asked him why, he said I didn't need to. I'd travel all the way to Bidston on the Wirral, which is a nightmare journey thinking 'why am I travelling all this way for just one hour?' What I later realised is that the old adage was true – it's quality and not quantity that counts.

I realised that, clear as diamonds in my eyes, when I went to Australia.

That was my first tournament since I'd started working with Phil.

The Australian Open was a round robin event and my main rival was Hunter from Canada. True to form, this turned out to be a tough match that went to another three-set tiebreak. Hunter had seven match points against me. So you could say it was in the stars that I was going to win the tournament.

You don't see the improvement yourself. It's only when you get to a tournament you realise how you've developed.

Phil Leighton *recalls*

It was different for me to coach Mark because he was the first wheelchair tennis player that I had taught. I'd always worked with able-bodied players before.

On his day, Mark was unbeatable in the world. He was a good learner and easy to deal with as he was so self-motivated. The coach's role is to motivate but Mark was already motivated, though there would be times where I would have to pick him up a little bit. He had confidence in me and I had confidence in him. Coaching him was very enjoyable.

THAILAND TRIUMPH

I found out I was Britain's first ever World No 1 in Thailand in February 2002. I had won the second of my Australian Open titles and Chris Johnson (Johnno) and me were on our way home. We went to Bangkok for a few days, I checked my e-mail at the hotel. There it was.

I was World No 1, one point above Draney. I was delighted. I couldn't believe it. The first British tennis player, at any level, to be World No 1.

Now that's what I call service to wheelchair tennis.

There can never, ever be another first British player ever to be

World No 1, because that was me, and the job's done, end of story.

I phoned home to tell my family but they already knew. I think everybody knew before I did. It was a bit of a surprise because, before Australia, I thought I could close the gap on Draney but I did not expect to overtake him. I held the top spot, the best Quad tennis player on the planet, for the next 14 months.

Chris Johnson (Johnno) – *Tennis teammate and roommate*

I was with Mark in Thailand when he found out he was World No 1. He was well chuffed! As a teammate I have to say he was a miserable git. He never smiled much. No, I'm joking.

A lot of people did say he was miserable, but I've shared a room with him for about four or five years and I've seen a different side to him where he can have a good laugh.

As a player, he had it mentally, which helps a lot. I hope he becomes a millionaire because then I might get to see a bigger smile on his face. He still wouldn't be happy, I sometimes think, if he was a millionaire.

Now, I know Johnno is joking because we shared a room for a few years and he is a really close mate, but I am fully aware that a lot of people on the tour thought I was miserable. I wasn't, I was just focused on playing and winning.

You see, the ones who thought I was miserable didn't know me, and they were also the ones that used to get knocked out in the first round and so could relax and have a holiday for the remaining days of the tournament.

But when you regularly make it to finals you have to remain focused and concentrated on your performance for the whole of the week. I rarely got knocked out first round so I rarely had chance to relax and have a bit of a jolly, like some I could mention, including a few coaches.

STRINGING VICTORIES TOGETHER

In 2002, I had a string of victories, first winning the Sydney Open and then the Australian Open. After Oz, it was time for the Florida Open, and another first place, beating Wagner in the final, followed by beating Van Erp in the final of the Belgian Open. But then I came down with gastroenteritis and lost the final of the British Open to Tachibana. I'm not making excuses, but I was bursting for the toilet throughout that match. Sorry to be indelicate, I did actually shit myself in the final – and it wasn't down to nerves.

I still only lost in a third set tiebreak though. Apart from that, no one could get anywhere near me; at the time, I was unbeatable.

It subsequently turned out that Tachibana had been exaggerating his disability and he was kicked out of the division. He wore a glove, but when his hands were looked at, they were a lot more functional than people thought. It surprised me because he was a nice bloke.

He wasn't the only player to be kicked out the division; there have been a few. The Quad division was originally created for players who had dysfunction in three or more limbs and so couldn't compete in the open division.

In the early days a few people would ridicule the division; however, when the division finally gained Paralympic status, was included in the World Team Cup, started to receive prize money and got its own world ranking, you began to get a load of mercenaries who were getting their arses kicked in open division, suddenly keen to join.

I still think there are players competing in the Quad division who contradict everything that the division was created for.

Unfortunately, due to the classification situation in disability sports, there are always going to be those who push the rules to the limit.

One of the faults in my game, and it is a big fault, is that once I've achieved what I've set out to achieve, I can take my eye off the ball a little.

In October 2002, I went to the US Open with one thing on my

mind. I knew that if I got further than Wagner in the tournament I would end the year as World Number One, and this was my main priority. In hindsight it was a ridiculous mindset to have going in to a major tournament. I achieved my goal as Wagner lost in the semi and I got to the final.

In the final I played Nick Taylor who I admire as a tennis player. He has achieved so much in spite of the severity of his disability. Nick was born with his disability, which has left him having to use an electric wheelchair as he has severe dysfunction in both arms.

He played a blinder and beat me fair and square. That's something that niggles me a little. I would love to have won America's biggest tournament.

Because I had switched off a little mentally, I lost the only US Open final I made it to. I was gutted; I think this occurred because I am very goal orientated and when I set a goal and achieve it, subconsciously I think the job is done. Then I relax. It was a ridiculous attitude to have and I paid dearly for it at the US Open.

What was quite interesting, though, was that after the match every American I spoke to, even the tournament referee, told me they wanted me to win.

We defended the World Team Cup title in Italy in September 2002. I lost my singles match to Wagner even though I had match point, and so the tie went down to the doubles. After the singles match there was a twenty-minute break before the doubles decider. I went to the toilet. As I passed a group of Americans, I heard one of them say, 'Eccleston's choked.'

Some idiots just don't know what they are talking about. Some loser who had never reached a final in their life, or was still being breast fed by his mummy, probably said this. I was fuming. If I had found out who had said it, I would have given them a piece of my mind.

I tried to get back on court for the final but the security guard wouldn't let me on; he said I had to have a ticket. I tried to explain that there wouldn't be a final without me as I was in it!!

I eventually convinced him and we played Wagner and Studwell in the doubles, winning 7–5, 7–6. This was the kind of environment I thrived on; a team situation where bottle mattered and I knew I had to take control in the tie break for us to retain the title.

We won and the place erupted. We had just won two World Team Cups in a row.

I went over to the area of the crowd where I had heard the 'choked' comment and screamed at them, 'Now who's a fucking choker?'

I received a number of messages of congratulations from high-ranking members of the wheelchair tennis community, which commented on how I had grabbed the match by the scruff of the neck.

The reason I performed so well in doubles and in World Team Cups was that I came from a team sport background and I enjoyed being part of a team.

James Pankhurst, *Great Britain coach, recalls*

Mark was a big time team player; in events like the World Team Cup he was very good. The time that was really shown and he stood up to the plate was the first year we won the World Team Cup in 2001. He was our number one player and he had the edge in all the tight matches. When we retained the title the following year, although he lost his singles match, in the doubles tiebreak he was unbelievable. It was great to see that. The light was closing in, Pete Norfolk was pretty tired and Mark was the one who pulled them through. Also in the doubles in the Paralympics against the Dutch when they were match point down, Mark saved two match points.

Rick Draney *also remembers*

I would rate Mark's skills as a tennis player in several different categories. Athletically, Mark was above average in skill and ability for a quad of his level of spinal cord injury. He was adept at maximizing what physical abilities he had and understood how to use what he had and make it work for him. Physically, I always felt I had a bit of an edge whenever we played in warmer conditions – he didn't sweat and

I did (most quads don't sweat – I got a lucky break, so to speak). Also, I was quite serious about my physical conditioning. I know Mark was, too but I think he had a tough time putting down the Pringles can. The longer a match went on, the more I felt I had an edge. His heart was his greatest asset. I don't know too many players that were (or are) more passionate about competing and desirous of winning than Mark, at least outwardly. Mark wore his heart on his sleeve – this is not to say that it was a good thing or a bad thing – only to say that it was obvious how competitive Mark was. Emotionally, Mark was challenged. I don't mean that in a demeaning way. It was Mark's fluctuating ability to keep his emotions in check early on that was his greatest challenge. A line call he didn't like, a distraction from the crowd, a missed shot and the like would often cause him to lose focus. He would vent his frustrations in various 'displays of displeasure' during a match, and sometimes allow it to carry over through a tournament. When he would do this, I 'knew' that I had him. It wasn't until he learned how to channel that frustration, to keep his emotions in check and regain his composure and focus while still playing with passion, that he achieved his greatest successes. Ultimately, his results speak for themselves as to how I (or anyone) would rate him as a tennis player.

I would like to think that any respect I may have 'earned' from Mark (or anyone else) was a result of my character, conduct, and integrity on and off the court. In Mark's case, it may also have something to do with the fact that I was involved in introducing him to the game and that I helped to inspire him to pursue it. Maybe it had something to do with a standard of achievement I had acquired and that he looked towards. Also, I think it has to do with rivalry. When you are No 1 or striving to be No 1, anyone who gets in your way and with whom you battle, over and over, becomes a rival. The fiercely competitive nature we both possessed fuelled that rivalry. Most people think that rivals hate (or have to hate) each other. In my opinion, rivals may hate to lose to each other, but really do respect one another in many ways – they recognize in someone else a similar desire to win, a tough competitor, an equal, if you will. Rivals may not necessarily be friends, but they can't help but respect a worthy opponent. Whatever the reasons Mark may have for respecting me, I respect what he *accomplished as an athlete and admire whatever he may do to encourage others.*

I have been blessed and feel very fortunate to have achieved on-court success in both tennis and rugby, and I am personally quite pleased with my results. I am humbled to think that Mark describes me as the greatest tetraplegic athlete of all time. There are many people who helped, influenced, and inspired me along the way, and they deserve credit for their part in my success. Mark was one of those people. He pushed me, motivated me, virtually forced me to be a better player because I ALWAYS wanted to beat him, just as he ALWAYS wanted to beat me.

I didn't spend as much time off the court with Mark as some of the other quad tennis players. I know there are plenty of stories to tell which no doubt area featured elsewhere in this book. I can't recall any specifics, even though I know we shared some laughs. I remember getting a chuckle or two at some of Mark's 'discussions' with a chair umpire or lines person – not so much that what he said was funny, but more along the lines of me laughing and saying to myself, 'Ha, ha, I've got you now!' We used to give Mark some good-natured ribbing about his 'frugality' (dare I say Mark was a bit of a tight wad?).

STARS IN THEIR EYES

In 2002, I got a letter from the BBC asking if I wanted to attend the Northwest Sports Personality of the year dinner. I was delighted, as I knew a lot of top sports stars would be there. Despite being World No 1 and the fact we'd just won our second World Team Cup, I didn't think for a minute that I would pick up the disabled personality of the year award. I thought the invite was just in recognition of the great year I'd had.

You've got your usual suspects when it comes to awards in the North-West; predictably enough, they were all up for the award.

I wasn't in danger of being star struck, though there were plenty of stars around. On my table was a famous sprinter who has got to be in the top three all-time biggest muppets I have ever met. He was right up his own arse. Someone involved with the BBC came over to him and asked if he would be happy to present an award. Let's just say he wasn't too pleased but he eventually, ever so kindly, agreed to do so. What I have generally found with track and field athletes is that they can be arrogant and feel that they are a cut above the rest – other athletes have said the same about them. Super-sprint then rang his agent and started complaining about having to present an award. And he wasn't being funny, like I was when I complained about the torture of doing a photo shoot with Kelly Brook!

I turned round to him and asked him if he was going to do it or not. He said he would. To which I replied, 'Good, please do shut up then.'

I'll give you another example of track and field arrogance. I was training for Athens at the Sportcity complex. They had a fitness conditioner who worked with the Great Britain basketball team and myself. It was very hard work. Two of you had to do a 200-metre sprint, then the other two would do it; when they finished, you started sprinting again and so on. You did six in total. You took a three-minute rest between sprints. This high jump coach came over to us and asked if we could stop doing this as there was a girl practicing the high jump and it was distracting her. I asked the coach if the girl was going to the Olympics? He said no. I then told him to do one, because I was bound for the games.

One of the women from the BBC came over to me at the awards and asked if the ramp leading onto the stage was too steep. I knew then that I was going to get the award. The ramp was very steep. When you look at the video now, it's obvious I have to give it some serious effort to get up there. When I first saw the ramp, I thought there's no way I am asking someone to push me up it; my mates will give me grief about it for years.

I was delighted to win. Receiving my award from the former Liverpool player, Steve McMahon, made it all the more special. It was nice to be appreciated even though they spelt my name wrong on the award!

Chapter 14

Going Downhill

In the beginning of 2003 the British Tennis Foundation decided that nobody was to go to Australia. I think this was partly due to finances and also with one eye on the qualification period for Athens. As I had won Sydney and the Australian Open in 2002, their decision meant I would lose a lot of points, since I wouldn't be defending the titles, but I was still World No 1.

The first major tournament we were allowed to enter was the Florida Open in April. This was when the 12 month qualification period for the Athens Paralympics began. I didn't have the best of preparations as only a couple of weeks before my Dad suffered a heart attack. I just didn't want to leave for the US. And it wasn't just because of Dad but also around this time, I began to feel something was wrong with me. I started to get pins and needles down my right arm and persistent niggles in my shoulder.

I got to Florida and played my first match. I did okay, but just didn't feel like myself. It was here that Pete Norfolk's wife started videoing me, something I found a bit strange because she had never done this before.

I made it through to the quarter-finals but lost to Pete Norfolk. That defeat ended my 14 month unbroken reign as World No 1.

I continued to train but the pins and needles and niggles in my shoulder just wouldn't go away. I didn't tell anyone. In hindsight, I think I was in denial as this was during the Paralympic qualification period and I did not want to jeopardise my chances in any way.

By the time we got to World Team Cup in Poland in June

2003, I was really struggling. I told the team management about my injury but did not tell them the full extent of how badly it was affecting me.

Our first match was against Israel. Again I was No 1. I played Weinberg, lost the first set, ended up down 5–2 in the second, yet I somehow still won. I didn't have any game plan as I was literally just flinging my racket about because I was so sore.

We then played Sweden and, again, I won my match, but it went on longer than it should have. The next match was against Holland. I lost my singles, but we won the doubles decider. This meant we made it to the final. Our opponents were the USA, coached by Jason Harnett, the man whose main specialty was getting people to beat me. I think by this time everyone knew I was carrying an injury because I was losing or struggling against players who, frankly, I should have been beating comfortably.

Pete Norfolk won the first singles match against Taylor. I then played Wagner. Although I played well in parts I was nowhere near 100% and lost. So we had to play a doubles decider. This is where I really needed Pete to take the game by the scruff of the neck and carry me through.

We lost.

I hid the extent of my injury in Poland. It was so bad that I didn't have a single bath during the two weeks we were there, as I couldn't lift myself into the water. I was struggling even to get out of bed. Every time I moved my shoulder I was in agony.

After the final I spoke to Jason in some depth. He was almost apologetic; he knew what bad shape I was in and said that my performance wasn't a reflection of my true ability. I hadn't been the Mark Eccleston he had known for the last few years. He was aware that I was injured and, so, as everything's fair in wheelchair tennis, he had told Wagner and Draney that three out of every four balls had to be hit to me. I feel he was uncomfortable doing that. But it was his job to win the team cup for the United States.

Jason is the only coach who consistently knew how to beat me. He always got his tactics spot on. It's no coincidence that whenever we beat the United States in a competition, Jason was not coaching them.

TEAM PLAYERS AND OTHERS

Certain people are just not team players and are driven to succeed purely on an individual basis. I'm a born and bred Rugby League lad. I'm into the team ethos. Even if you don't get on with someone in your team, you do what has to be done as you are all singing from the same hymn sheet.

After Poland, I felt very guilty as I had played with an injury and felt I had let the team down, so I sent a text to the other team members apologizing.

I am more than happy to take the credit when I play well and I am also man enough to take the responsibility when I play poorly, I didn't play well and because of that we lost, so I apologised. Not everyone I sent the text to replied back, which pissed me off a little.

After Poland, I played in France and told a physio that my shoulder was bad. She gave me the following advice – just lie down, and it will be okay.

Are you having a laugh?

I couldn't get a bath or get out of bed without it causing me major grief, and she was telling me to just have a 'lie down'.

I was playing tournaments and being knocked out first round. In France I finally admitted to myself that there was something seriously wrong and I needed to get it sorted.

My lottery funding gave me access to services within the English Institute of Sport. In August 2003 I went to see a physio by the name of Matt Lancaster. He identified the problem straight away.

Matt found that I exhibited limited cervical change, hypo-mobility throughout the mid and low cervical right articular pillar. When he conducted neurodynamic tests and active trigger points through the muscles in this region, it reproduced the tingling in my arm. He thought that the symptoms probably suggested a low cervical radiculopathy along with associated secondary trigger points. The treatment was gentle mobilisation of the cervical spine, trigger point release along with acupuncture, mesotherapy and neurodynamic mobilisation.

To make the above paragraph easier for duffers like me; he found where the problem was, he was able to reproduce the problem and, therefore, able to treat it.

I went to the Institute twice a week from August to the beginning of October where Matt would do his thing. But it wasn't all treatment.

Once he began to talk about football. He then shouted over to the next cubicle asking the occupants their opinion on me being a Liverpool fan. The girl on the other side proceeded to make known her utter contempt for anything to do with Liverpool. It turns out she was a Man United fan so I went on a ten-minute tirade. First, I ranted that women know absolutely nothing about football. Then, I went on to say that women who support Man United should be jailed.

I asked Matt who the girl was and he wouldn't tell me due to, in his words, patient confidentiality. It turns out she was Tracey Neville, twin sister of Phil Neville. I told Matt I was so happy he hadn't asked me my opinion on the Nevilles because I would have really upset her then.

Matt Lancaster – *lead physiotherapist London Region, English Institute of Sport*

Mark was pretty down about where he was at in terms of his tennis, and his shoulder was obviously the major cause of concern. He was clearly focused on the Athens Paralympics, and the chance to compete for a medal was still driving him strongly.

Mark had pain in his shoulder, but of greater concern was the sensation of pins and needles, which extended all the way down his arm. Clearly it was not a simple 'shoulder injury', and there was a degree of nerve irritation involved.

The difficulty with Mark's shoulder was that it wasn't a purely 'sporting injury'. It was probably related to his disability as much as his sport. If he didn't have the disability or if he didn't play wheelchair tennis, it might not have emerged as a problem and obviously there was a limited amount that could be done to change his disability. To compound things, it was exacerbated not just by his sport, which is often the case with able-bodied athletes, but by everyday activities such as driving his car or pushing his wheelchair. As a result it was harder to 'rest' the injury and allow it to recover fully. Interestingly it was not his dominant shoulder (the one he holds the racquet with) but his other arm, which was hugely important for propelling his wheelchair.

What was he like to work with? Up and down. His shoulder settled reasonably quickly with treatment, but it was clear that he still had a number of hurdles to overcome before he returned to the level of tennis he had been playing prior to the injury.

His vocal supporting of Liverpool sometimes got in the way of his treatment because he wouldn't bloody shut up about the Reds.

HINDSIGHT IS ALWAYS WISE

By late September I was feeling much, much better. Then it was off to America to compete in three tournaments, which in hindsight was a huge mistake. I started off playing well, and had physiotherapy on a daily basis.

The first tournament was at Hilton Head. I played Pete in the semis. I played really well, losing a close match. Again I noticed during the match that his wife had filmed the game. I asked her afterwards for a copy of it and she said she would provide me with one.

I never received it.

After the match one of the players spoke to me and told me that people had been writing me off and saying I was finished. Kick a man when he is down, eh?

The second tournament was in Alabama. I didn't perform particularly well, but I did manage to reach the semi-final. After the game, though, the problems in my shoulder and arm flared up again.

By the time of the US Open in San Diego in 2003, my shoulder was hurting as much as it had been before I started going to see Matt at the English Institute of Sport. It was so sore that it had to be taped up. I struggled to even hit the ball. I faced my good friend, Lev from Israel, in the first round and, as I couldn't play properly, he beat me in three sets.

It was in San Diego that Pete Norfolk started ignoring me. He would push past and not speak. I won't say it upset me, but I was surprised. I spoke to one of the Great Britain team staff. They said that I was not to take it personally as he was not really talking to anybody. It was bizarre. At the end of the US Open, I pulled Pete over and asked him if he had a problem with me. He told me he didn't but he was sick of people questioning whether he should be in the division.

Pete said he just wanted to play his matches and go. I told him I had never questioned his right to be in the division, although, in fact, I had done so privately. He told me he would give me a ring the week after and discuss what we would do for Athens.

He never called.

When I came back, I told Matt it was a mistake to have done three tournaments in a row and he agreed with me. I think I had risen to about No 14 in the rankings, as I had fallen as low as No 20 in the previous months.

Matt Lancaster *recalls*

He had a flare up not long after returning to the circuit after San Diego, and this set him back quite a bit, mentally. He probably just wasn't ready to play so intensely that early on. The shoulder settled reasonably quickly, but driving his car continued to produce pins and needles for some time, even when he was back and playing well. He was a pretty positive athlete to deal with, by and large, and his focus on Athens was admirable, but he certainly went through periods of doubt as to whether he'd make it. As a physiotherapist, helping him to manage those expectations and negative beliefs was probably a bigger challenge that settling his shoulder down.

TOP TEN

We were all under the impression that to qualify for Athens in the Quad division we had to be ranked amongst the world's top sixteen players. Wrong. Six months into the qualification period, The British Paralympic Association informed us that we had to be in the top ten to go to the Olympics. Why they only told us this then is one of life's little mysteries.

I began to see Matt again twice weekly. In November I went to Nottingham knowing I had to do well as I needed to move up four places to get into the top 10. I played really well and beat Hunter who was No 3 in the world at the time, and then went on to beat Draney in the final. I went to Prague in December and won there as well. But I still wasn't guaranteed a place in Athens.

Chapter 15

Lead up to Athens

In early 2004 we went to Australia. I knew a good performance in Sydney or Melbourne would ensure qualification for the 2004 Athens Paralympics.

I beat Hunter in the quarter-final of the Sydney Open. During this match, Pete Norfolk's wife again reappeared with her video camera. I asked her to stop pointing it straight at me, but she refused. The tournament referee told me there was nothing he could do, except ask her to move back because she was leaning over the fence.

In the semi-final I played Pete Norfolk. James Pankhurst, the Great Britain coach, totally blew the situation. He told us that because he was our coach he couldn't warm either of us up, which was fair enough. Another Great Britain coach offered his services but Pankhurst insisted that none of our coaches should be involved. That was fine with me; I would sort out my own training partner.

Next morning I arrived at the tennis centre. To my absolute amazement Norfolk was warming up with another Great Britain coach, who, coincidentally, is a left-hander, same as me and has an alarm clock that doesn't work.

I went absolutely nuts. I played well in the match but lost. Afterwards, I went mad at Pankhurst and I think he realised he had messed up, big time. I was later told that Pete was unhappy with James' decision not to allow British coaches to warm us up. I firmly believe that, at this stage, the British Tennis Foundation saw Pete as their best chance of a gold medal in Athens and so he was allowed to get away with a little bit more.

I didn't play doubles in Sydney because I wanted to concentrate on my singles and getting enough points. Getting to the semi-final would more or less guarantee I would qualify for Athens. We then went down to Melbourne and I was under the impression that I would be playing doubles with Pete. All our main competitors who would be in Athens were there, so it made sense – it did to me anyway.

Anybody would have thought that, in Paralympic year, Pete and me would play together. However, on arriving in Melbourne I was informed that Pete did not want to play doubles with me, a decision I found staggering. He eventually played doubles with Roy Humphries, another British player who was close to qualifying via the wild card system. In my opinion this decision was made by the British Tennis Foundation in the hope that Roy and Pete would do well and Roy's double ranking would rise, strengthening his chances of getting the wildcard.

Because I was only told Pete wasn't playing doubles with me at such a late stage there was nobody else available to be my partner, as all the other players were paired off. It was only because of an injury to Draney the morning the tournament started that I got to play with Wagner. This was quite ironic as we went on to beat Pete and Roy in the final, which tickled me somewhat, as you can imagine.

In the singles I played the best tennis I had played in a long time during the quarters where I beat Bas Van Erp. Again, I was to play Pete in the semis.

The night before the match I was in bed and my scouse roommate, Jamie came in; it was one of those situations where the more he tried to be quiet the more noise he made. The next thing he is jumping up and down at the window screaming in the broadest scouse accent you can imagine. 'Eccy! Look at this lar!'

I wanted to know what was going on, as I wasn't impressed about being woken up. He told me that across the way he could clearly see into another room. Inside that room a gentleman and his lady friend were participating in adult activities. Needless to say I was out of that bed before he'd finished the sentence and went to the window. Across the courtyard, I could see into the room and, no shagging doubt, there was sexual activity of a very entertaining and explicit nature on display.

Jamie said, 'I knew this would happen, it's Valentine's Day. I knew someone would have to be shagging.'

I saw the wisdom of his line of thought.

I told him to go down and along the corridor so he could get the room number and we could phone them up. He went down, got the room number and came back. We rang them up. I could see the young gentleman answer the phone, but what was impressive was his concentration. He picked the phone up without breaking stride.

Jamie drew a mental blank at this point and asked, 'Is Johnno there?' I couldn't believe this was the best he could come up with.

I looked through the curtains to see the lad still going for glory with his female companion. He had hung up the phone and then started dialling. I immediately thought that he was going to ring reception and find out which room had just rung him. Then, he was going to track us down and kill us.

I thought I'd head down to reception.

It was about 2.30 in the morning. The house phone was on a desk by a sofa filled with six Japanese players.

'Arigato' (I speak a bit of the lingo).

I picked up the phone and rang the room again.

He was an Aussie and asked me what I wanted.

I started saying. 'GO ON MY SON.'

He started saying it back to me.

I was now shouting down the phone. 'GO ON MY SON.'

He too was shouting, 'GO ON MY SON.'

The next thing all the Japanese started shouting, 'GO ON MY SON.'

It was hilarious and I was laughing that much I had to put the phone down.

I went back to the room and Jamie asked me what I had been saying to him. I asked why and he said because the lad was on top of his lady friend with the phone in one hand and pumping his other fist in the air.

The next morning we went down for breakfast and we were telling this story. As we were doing so, the Japanese group came in and they went off again with cries of 'Go on my son'. We had never been able to clearly see the faces of the two people having fun in their room. There was however one bloke with a girl on the next table. As he left the room he looked over at me and winked.

And just in case you want to know about the tennis. Pete Norfolk had beaten me pretty convincingly the week before and, although he beat me again here, I played a lot better. My qualification for Athens was assured.

VIDEO NASTIES

In April 2004 I went back to Florida. I had been having regular physio with Matt and was feeling pretty good. However, in every one of my matches, Pete Norfolk's wife was videoing me again. It was really getting on my nerves. I felt it was an inappropriate, because she was head physio for the British Paralympic Association (BPA), the organisation which ultimately decided who was selected for the Paralympics.

So here you had the head physio of the BPA videoing me. Obviously she would be taking that film home to study my weaknesses and how to beat me.

Oh and she just also happened to be the wife of my main competitor and teammate. What would have happened if I needed treatment in Athens and our tennis physio was away treating someone else? The head physio of the BPA would be responsible for my treatment. This was a clear conflict of interest, or so I thought.

Back to Florida: she claimed that she was videoing everyone, but I argued otherwise. My point was proven in the doubles final. After what happened in Melbourne it was agreed that Pete and I would play doubles in tournaments that we both entered during the lead up to Athens.

We played together in Florida and in the final we faced the Americans, who would be our main opposition in Athens.

Nobody videoed the final. I would have thought if you were playing your main competition for a gold medal in a final then that would be an ideal match to video.

What annoyed me even more was the Great Britain management's insistence that Pete's wife was doing nothing wrong and that I was being paranoid. However, when the sports psychologist from the British Paralympics Association saw what was going on, he agreed that I had a point.

He was also correct in telling me that I should rise above this and ignore it, and I probably would have but for the way in which certain members of the British Tennis Foundation dealt with the situation.

It finally came to an explosive head at the British Open in July. I got to the quarter-final where I played Bas Van Erp. Phil Leighton, my coach, had come down to watch. He was already aware of what had gone on with regards to the videoing. Needless to say, filming was taking place so I shouted up to James Pankhurst, asking him to resolve the situation.

Even Phil, who is so laid back that the man is downright horizontal, was furious and taken aback by the aggression showed by certain people.

Phil Leighton – *Mark's coach*

There were some personality clashes within the camp. People definitely worked against Mark. I talked to him about this at the time. It's only normal when you're at the top that others will try to pull you down.

I arrived at the conclusion, rightly or wrongly, that Pete's wife was just doing it to disrupt my game and piss me off. I played terribly in the match and lost it. I was fuming at this stage.

Dawn Newbury, the Great Britain team manager, had now joined Pankhurst in the stands. I pushed over to them and

173

shouted up, 'If you want a doubles medal in Athens, fucking sort this out because you lot mean fuck all to me.'

Ten minutes after coming off court, I got the word that the British Tennis Foundation management wanted a word with me. The next day a meeting was called.

I went up, entered the room and faced four high-ranking members of my sport's governing body.

I was met first thing with the words, 'Mark, it has come to our attention that you used foul and abusive language yesterday and we're horrified that the Mayor of Nottingham was in earshot of this. Thankfully he didn't hear this because, if he had, it could have had serious repercussions.'

They asked me to repeat what I had said.

So, I did, gladly.

I was told that they were not very impressed at all with me saying they didn't mean that much to me. I told them I was not impressed with the way I had been treated these last few months. Then, what I regard as the real reason this meeting was called, was introduced into the conversation.

They said that Pete had also heard my outburst and was upset as he thought I had a problem with playing doubles with him in Athens.

I had been on at them for months about an issue that was affecting me and they had done absolutely nothing. Then he gets upset because I swear and it's a major incident.

I was fuming. I was so upset that I stormed out the room. I eventually calmed down and went back in.

It was then suggested that a meeting be called in which Pete was present. I was to explain that I had no problem playing doubles with him and that I was also to apologise to him!

They asked me if I wanted the meeting that day or the next. There was no way I was hanging around there for another day so I said I would like to get it over with.

Half an hour later I went back up. To my absolute horror the same four officials were there, as well as Pete, his coach and his wife!

So now there were seven of them and just little old me.

It felt like I was in front of a firing squad.

I began by telling Pete that I did not have any problem playing doubles with him but I was upset at his wife filming me. She said she filmed all the players but I just didn't want to know by this point. I then apologised to everyone for the foul language I had used.

Everyone accepted my apology except his wife who said: 'I hear your apology and acknowledge your apology but I don't accept your apology, because let's face it, Mark, what you say and what you do are two different things. I would like to see an improvement in your behaviour.'

I nearly fell through the fucking floor!

Even Dawn Newbury showed some bottle and asked what she meant by that. I left feeling bullied and upset. In fact, I was so upset I was in no fit state to drive home.

I had just been through the most embarrassing and humiliating experience of my life.

James Pankhurst came running out after me and he too was clearly upset. He said something to me that I will always be grateful to him for, but the damage had been done. I knew there and then that, as soon as Athens was done, that was it; I didn't want any more to do with some of those that were in that room.

About a week later my girlfriend, Lucy, asked if anyone from the British Tennis Foundation had contacted me to see how I was and if I got home okay. I didn't hear a thing, which I thought was an absolute disgrace considering the treatment I got and the emotional state I left the meeting in.

Chapter 16

The Drugs Test

Prior to Athens we had a team get together in Southampton to go over media issues and the procedures we would follow during the games. Privately I approached the British Paralympics Association doctor, along with the Great Britain team manager, expressing my concerns regarding any physio treatment that I might require. After the way I was treated in Nottingham I did not want to receive treatment from certain individuals. Both the doctor and Dawn Newbury told me that wouldn't happen. Other promises were made that, true to form, turned out to be a load of bullshit as well.

During this team get together, the Great Britain Tennis physio came in and said that she was sorry to spring this on us, but we all had to go for a drugs test. We all trekked up to the testers' room in pairs.

I went up with Simon Hatt, a really funny bloke. We were taking the piss out of the testers, big time. Every day drugs testers must hear 'Are you taking the piss?'

You had to fill a form in stating what medication you had taken in the past seven days. I didn't put anything down as my mind had gone blank. I went back downstairs and suddenly remembered I had taken Viagra a couple of days earlier.

I went up to the physio and told her what I had taken and that I'd not put it on the form. She took me back upstairs where I told them about the Viagra. They put it on the form; I went back downstairs again.

I asked the physio, 'Do I have to put everything on the form?' She confirmed that I did.

I said, 'What about that cream you gave me for the rash on my leg?' Her face immediately drained of all colour, she looked like Casper the Friendly Ghost with anaemia.

She said, 'Mark, I'd forgot about that ... it's banned.' I went back up to the tester and told them about the cream. The physio was panicking – and so was I.

The cream had hydrocortisone in it and cortisone is a banned substance. She went to speak to the Chief Medical Officer at the British Olympic Committee who confirmed it was banned, but there was good news. For it to show up in my bloodstream I would have had to have a bath in it day and night for about eight weeks.

However, there was a slim chance it could have got into my system, and if that was the case, no Athens for Mark. Instead, I'd get a two year ban.

It usually takes four weeks for a drugs test result to come through but you can pay for it to be done in about five days. I paid and it came back clear.

Chapter 17

Athens 2004

Just before Athens, a friend of mine got married and I really wanted to go to the wedding, but I was playing in the Swiss Open. I asked the tournament director if I reached the doubles final, could it be moved to an earlier time? He said it was okay by him if the other players agreed. I lost my singles semi-final against Wagner and then won my doubles semi. After that, it was straight back out to play the doubles final, which we lost. I was knackered, and it was a very hot day, too. But I made the wedding that night.

In one day I played three tennis matches, got from Geneva to St Helens, had the three S's (s**t, shower, shave) and made it to the wedding by 9 p.m.

Not bad eh?

Bet Henman has never done that.

And there I had my final beer before trying for Paralympic glory.

The facilities in Athens were fantastic. I had been on a 'recce' in April 2004 and had my doubts about the venue. All the stadiums looked half-built, at best. The Paralympics were in September and I thought 'there is no way this is going to be ready'. They got it done though, to be fair. A lot of it was touch up jobs and covering things with sheets, but they did it. I was very impressed with the set up. Like everyone else, I was expecting something to go wrong. The Paralympics are supposed to be the pinnacle of your career and I had worried that they would be a farce like Atlanta. The Greeks pulled it off, though.

Having said that, I didn't like the rooming arrangements at the games. Eight in an apartment is not my idea of fun. You're going to get that, though, wherever the Paralympics are held. It's just something you have to prepare for psychologically. You're screwed if you don't. I had done Atlanta so I knew what was coming. Even so, it was hard to cope with ten days of it. Sport isn't just physically demanding – it puts you under great mental strain as well.

Competing, what you do on the court, is only part of what you have to do well. It drains you to be away from home, and in such weird surroundings. Our apartment was right at the back of the village and the food hall was at the front – with a few hills in between. A bus came round picking athletes up, but it was always full; by the time the next one came round you could have pushed there in your chair. It was a ten minute push, which I often did. But doing that time and again, day after day, caught up with me by the end of the week.

I always remember the opening ceremony at Atlanta. Brian Worrall said he wasn't going. I asked him why and he said he had already done one. It is a long, drawn out, boring event until you enter the stadium, he said, but added that as I hadn't seen one before, I should go.

I went and I agreed with his assessment. You're sat outside the stadium for three or four hours because every country has to parade and be announced to the crowd. It's boring, until your turn comes to go in to the arena.

The opening ceremony in Athens was a few days before the tennis started. If it had been the night before our competition, I don't think I would have entertained it, as it would have disrupted my preparation too much. But I went. It was an amazing experience.

There was the transition from being bored to buzzing after entering a stadium full of 80,000 people. It was a massive leap psychologically, but also mentally draining. Once they light the torch, it is pretty good. You can't compete in the Paralympics and not do an opening ceremony.

I got the toughest singles draw imaginable. I was also concerned about the heat in Athens, but as all my matches were in the evening, it never became an issue. That was lucky, as the mid-day heat was scorching. I used the afternoons to practice, and could only manage twenty minutes on the court, because of my inability to sweat.

First up, I played Polidori from Italy who had beaten me only two weeks earlier, in Livorno. I started poorly and lost the first set.

I knew that if I didn't get my act together then I would be out of the tournament. However, I took the second set. He began to play nervously, so I went on to win the match.

That put me into the quarter final against Bas Van Erp.

Van Erp was always a very hit and miss sort of player – on form, he was incredible, but if he stumbled at all, his game might just disintegrate. He was on fire during the first set, and I couldn't get a look in losing 6–1. I fought back, taking the second set 6–3 after being 3–0 down, and we were all set up for an exciting finale.

It was an incredible match, and at 5–4 up in the third I had two match points on his serve.

Now, it was generally accepted that Van Erp was a bit of a choker. He had, on a number of occasions double faulted on match point against me.

Unfortunately not this time.

He hit an ace, then an unreturnable serve, and went on to win the match 6–1 3–6 7–5.

People have since asked me if I am upset about having had two match points in a Paralympics quarter final, and going on to lose.

The answer to that is – absolutely not.

Van Erp had the bottle to go for two big serves and they paid off. So full credit to the man, he deserved it.

I didn't lose that match: Bas Van Erp won it. It's as simple as that.

Now, if I had a clear shot at a winner and missed, then that would have haunted me for the rest of my life.

Van Erp went on to lose to Pete Norfolk in the semis, and

Pete then won the final against Wagner. In fact, Pete won every one of his single matches pretty easily. A staggering achievement, considering that just a couple of months earlier he had severely dislocated his shoulder.

LESS THAN 100%

Due to all my shoulder problems I stopped being the 100% Mark Eccleston in 2003 and, as a result, I was always playing catch-up.

I also don't believe the tennis played in Athens was the best the Quad division has ever seen. If the Rick Draney of the late '90s or the Mark Eccleston of the 2001 World Team Cup had showed up in Athens, the outcome would have been different.

However they didn't, Pete was the best player that particular week – so fair play to him.

In the doubles semi final against Holland we lost the first set and were 5–2, 40–15 down in the second, two match points away from losing and missing the chance to play in the Paralympic final.

However, we turned it around again. I feel we ended up with silver due to my efforts in that match. I just kept telling myself that I hadn't gone through all the shit of the past few years to get knocked out now. I was desperate to get to the final.

A crowd of about 8000 watched the doubles final. That was an amazing buzz seeing so many people turn up to watch us. As the USA had Taylor playing in his electric wheelchair, the neutrals in the crowd sided with them.

With a tennis venue, the crowd seem to be further away from you, whereas when playing rugby the crowd is right on top of you and the atmosphere is better. I've played in front of smaller crowds playing rugby, which had a better atmosphere than the Paralympic tennis finals, to be honest.

I got us through that semi-final, and spectators who were there that day have said the same. I wanted it so badly after all the grief I had been through. But in the final Pete was in a different place. He had got the one he really wanted, the one everyone wanted, the singles gold.

If Pete had lost the singles final, then I think we would have won the doubles. He now has a doubles silver medal because of me, and I have a silver medal because of him. I felt we both could have played better in the final although, yet again, Jason had got his tactics spot on.

I'm disappointed that from April 2003 onwards, I couldn't function the way I wanted to on court. Physically I just wasn't capable of it. It got to the point where I couldn't hit a cow's arse with a banjo, so I suppose winning a silver medal was a great achievement. Although at the time I didn't think so.

Winning a silver medal is a very strange feeling.

To get silver, you have to lose the final, and not just any old final either. A lot of people don't understand that. The commentators say, 'You've got the silver medal, what a great achievement.' However, I will guarantee you that every person who's up on that podium receiving a silver medal is feeling disappointed, or they should be.

The awards ceremony is usually within an hour of the event so you're still feeling sad that you have just lost. You're annoyed. If you look at the television coverage of me going up to receive the silver medal, you can see clearly I don't look happy. People who saw the interview I did with the BBC after the ceremony called me miserable. But you have to put yourself in my situation.

I had just lost a Paralympic final and, annoyingly, certain people within the Great Britain set up seemed happy with that. But I was absolutely gutted.

At the closing ceremony I told Jason Harnett my tennis career was just about over. He very kindly repeated his view that my Barcelona match with Draney was one of the best he had ever seen. It was some comfort.

There was also another reason I didn't look too happy at the closing ceremony, a reason I have never spoken about till now.

In the months leading up to the Paralympics two people close to me died.

One was my dad's brother, my Uncle Bill. He had been ill for a long time and eventually passed away in early May. I was playing in the National Championships at the time.

I phoned my Auntie up and told her I was going to leave the tournament and come and see her. I was pretty upset. All my grandparents had died when I was very young, so this was the first time, as an adult, I lost a close family member. She told me to play on, as that was what Uncle Bill would have wanted. However my heart wasn't in it to compete, and I left.

I just wanted to go and see her, then get home and see my dad.

The other person was Mike Dunne, brother of Stuart, from Cyclone. Mike was responsible for designing and building my wheelchairs. Whenever I had a new idea for my tennis chair he was the man I would go and see. He always made sure I was sorted out.

Prior to the final in Athens I had written the words 'BILL ECC & MIKE D: GONE BUT NOT FORGOTTEN' on the front of a T-shirt.

When the match had finished I put the T-shirt on. I intended to open my tracksuit top and show it to the cameras after the medal ceremony.

However one of the tournament officials saw that I had put it on and approached me. He told me that I was to keep my tracksuit zipped up and I was not to show my T-shirt to the cameras.

I told him to get out of my face.

This jobsworth then insisted I take it off or I wouldn't be allowed out to receive my medal.

What was I thinking about on the medal rostrum as I was listening to the American national anthem?

My dad and Stuart, two people who, earlier that year, had both lost brothers.

I dedicated the medal to them and to my Uncle Bill and Mike Dunne.

Some things are more important than a tennis match.

BBC BLUES

The media, and especially the BBC, are a pain. In the interview after the medal ceremony I mentioned that I was dedicating the medal to my Uncle Bill and Mike and asked if they would put that out with the interview. They said they would – and then they didn't.

But it was fine for them to pester me as soon as I was knocked out of the singles.

After the singles match they came over. I had literally just shook hands with Van Erp and I hadn't even got out of my tennis chair and they were pestering for me to go on camera.

I told them I would do it in a minute. The press officer from the British Paralympic Association then came over and said, 'When you said in a minute, did you mean literally a minute?'

Incredible!

This didn't impress me one little bit.

Yet they couldn't find the time to do me a favour and broadcast my dedication.

If I was a press officer with the British Paralympic Association and I had just seen a man get to match point in a game and then lose, I would wait a while before approaching him for an interview. She has obviously never played sport at élite level, or if she has, she has never lost an Olympic final.

I feel that media treatment of disability sport is, on the whole, poor. That said, it's better in the UK than in some other countries. The US is terrible for sure. They showed about one hour of the Paralympics on TV and that was about a year after the actual event.

The BBC did something on it every night, which was good. My problem is that they show the same sports and the same people every time. This was the first Paralympics where Britain won medals at tennis and it got very little coverage. Yet they show extended coverage of certain other sports over and over again.

They also concentrated heavily on one athlete who had been disqualified from her classification in athletics and on Tanni Grey

Thompson who got more coverage than tennis, for coming last in a race!

Such lack of coverage ignores the effort you have to make to qualify – 12 months of travelling the world and playing tournaments to get points. For other sports it's just a few minutes, which admittedly you have to train for. In swimming and track and field, for example, you have to achieve a set time or distance and that's it.

It would help if the BBC saw more to disabled sport than basketball, swimming and Tanni Grey Thompson.

It's a subject that winds a lot of wheelchair athletes up, but they'll only talk about it privately in case they get into trouble with the powers that be.

What a lot of people don't know is that, in swimming and track and field, due to the classification system, only four or five competitors may qualify in some classes. This means sometimes there needs only be one race between them to determine the medal winners. No first round, second round, quarters and semis for them to fight through.

My thinking is that certain people are in a position where they could push and promote all disability sports, but they don't. Now, as a coach, I will not do interviews to promote Mark Eccleston, but I will happily talk to the media about disability sport in general. There are so many other wheelchair athletes who have achieved great things – and yet no one has ever heard of them.

Mark's brother, Gary, *reflects*

Mark has not had the recognition he deserves and I think a lot of that has something to do with him coming from up North, whereas players from down South seem to get more press. When he did get recognition, though, it was great. I feel very proud of all his achievements, I have friends in the Manchester area and I'd be out with them and they'd tell me they'd seen Mark on TV, and wanted to know what he was up to.

Pat, *Mark's mum agrees*

He deserves recognition; he never got the publicity he deserved when he was playing. The national press was bad enough but the locals in St Helens didn't give him much coverage either. The way St Helens treated him was disappointing considering the Mayor of Wirral inducted Mark into the Wirral Sporting Hall of Fame and presented him with a certificate for excellence. He's never had anything from his home town. He was at the BBC Northwest Sports Personality of the year and when they announced his name and home town, someone from St Helens RLFC came over and said that he should be sat with them. They admitted that they had never heard of him before, though.

At first being interviewed on TV is quite exciting, but the more it happens, the duller it gets. They will sometimes tell you what to say before the camera comes on. The press photographers are worse, they want you to do corny poses and it takes ages for them to get the shots they want. How hard is it to take a photo? It's good to see yourself on telly, even though sometimes you feel a bit of a prune watching yourself.

HOME AGAIN

Initially the silver medal meant nothing to me and it only started to mean something to me when I got home and everyone wanted to see it. My mum, dad and brothers were ecstatic.

Pat

It was fantastic to see Mark win the silver medal in Athens, he worked really hard for it and he deserved it.

I put his success down to his guts and willpower and, also, he is the type of person who can't sit still. He always needs to be doing something and his mind is working overtime, all the time, for his next goal.

Gary

I feel very proud of all his achievements.

His drive and single mindedness have helped him achieve. To get to the top you have to have a bit about you. The best in any sport have that little extra about them; they know they're good at what they do.

He's done that and been a success at what he's been involved in. He's seen more of the world than I'll ever see through sport. I look back to what he was like after the accident and I didn't know whether he'd even be able to look after himself. If somebody had said to me then that he'd end up travelling around the world, I would have said 'no chance'.

Michael

Just before Mark got injured, I spoke with one of the leaders of the British Tennis Foundation; she said that Mark was a certainty for the final in singles – that's how well he was playing and how highly he was regarded at the time. I was going to go, then I wasn't, then I didn't. Something I now regret, although in some ways I don't – I wanted to see him win gold.

I know Mark's was initially disappointed for himself.

Given the lack of preparation leading-up to Athens, to win silver was a fantastic achievement.

His determination was probably the single biggest factor in achieving the medal. The other emotion is one of frustration. Athens came around at completely the wrong time for Mark. In approximately 18 months prior to his injury, Mark almost cleaned-up all over the world.

He achieved one of his goals in reaching the No 1 ranked position – the first Brit to do so. Life's full of 'ifs'.

If only Athens had come around when Mark was ranked No 1, then I am convinced he would have returned with two gold medals.

The difference between Mark and sports people who haven't achieved as much is that, while people have some of the following attributes, I don't know anyone who has them all. Determination, single minded-ness, focus, aggression (sometimes controlled, sometimes not – on court). Hates to lose. Confidence. Will power.

Dr Clive Glass – *Deputy Clinical Director, North West Regional Spinal Injuries Centre*

Mark went into the Paralympics having lost the World No 1 spot. But by concentrating on his strengths and remaining focused he achieved his success. In the singles he was beaten by a better player on the day and in the doubles he played to the best of his ability. He recognises that he could not have done any more and, on their day, any one of a number of players could win a championship. The important thing therefore is not to come out of a game thinking you have lost, but to leave any game knowing you have played your best. If someone raises their game more, you do not win, but you haven't lost either.

Matt Lancaster

Mark's effort to win a medal was fantastic because he had to overcome, not just the physical aspect of his injury, but everything else that went with it – self-doubt, altered training and preparation, and possibly fear...

Until I got home, I was gutted. Everyone who says that a silver medal is a great achievement has obviously never lost an Olympic or Paralympic final. It's a horrible experience. I hated it.

However, I take the medal into schools now and the kids are amazed by it and that means a lot to me. It brings a lot of joy to a lot of people and that is special.

At the end of the day, how many people can you bump into down the high street who have an Olympic or Paralympic medal?

Mr Soni, who had treated me when I was first injured at sixteen, came out to Athens. Running alongside the Paralympics was a convention for spinal injury consultants. We arranged to meet up for a drink. There in the middle of Athens was me, Lucy, Lucy's brother, James Pankhurst, the Great Britain coach, Mr Soni and another doctor called Pedro, who treated me with injections in the lead up to Athens. Obviously I am glad Lucy was there but I was also glad James Pankhurst was there because after a bit of a dodgy start, he eventually figured me out. He helped me a great deal during his time as coach especially in the lead up to Athens with all the shit I had to deal with.

I have a photo of me with Mr Soni holding my medal. It was a nice moment as things had come full circle. This man had been there when I came into hospital as a sixteen-year-old after my accident. Now we were having a beer together as we held my Paralympic medal aloft, pissed, in the middle of Athens.

James Pankhurst – *GB Tennis Coach*

It was an amazing thing to have a drink with Mark and his consultant in Athens. However, I got more pleasure out of the times I saw him absolutely excel on the court. The moments that stand out for me are the times where he won great matches at the US Open and in the singles and doubles at the Paralympics. There are some matches he lost that stand out, like in the Paralympics where he lost a very close singles match. After those defeats I would try to help him. The winning was very nice but seeing him excel on the court was a real pleasure.

It was a very good experience coaching Mark. It's a difficult sport and a difficult sport for Mark in that, in some respects, he had a greater disability than other players he was competing against. That made his achievements in his career even greater. It was a great pleasure working with him.

It's difficult to compare Mark with able-bodied players I've worked with; you don't know how any of them would cope with the trauma that Mark has been through. In terms of fighting spirit and bloody-mindedness there is no-one else to compare him with.

I never treated Mark as someone in a wheelchair and that's not the way he would want anyone to treat him. He wanted someone to treat him as the world class athlete he was.

If I think about the three years I worked with Mark, it wasn't really me who was taking the risk, it was Mark. I developed a good relationship with him and as my experience of coaching him developed, I saw that he'd done something extraordinary. Nobody else knows how they would cope with his situation. To actually come through the other side and become World No 1 and achieve what he's achieved – not just in tennis but also in other wheelchair sports – is something that humbles you.

We had plenty of disagreements over me telling him there were certain things he needed to do on court. I felt at times he would get too angry on court and I wanted him to be a bit calmer. Even after those things though, I would class him as a close friend. If you can spend the amount of time with somebody that I spent with Mark and still be close friends through some very difficult times, then that says a lot for him.

As I have said, I had a lot of problems with injuries and other issues in the lead up to the Athens Paralympics. Lucy's support and help at that time was unconditional and total. Without it I would have struggled big time. She kept me calm and encouraged me when I felt like chucking it all in. They do say you need to go through a load of bad apples to reach a good one. I certainly had a few bad apples in my time but that ended when I met her.

I sometimes think of certain moments during my career that were good, but I don't have to think too hard to realise that that moment in the middle of Athens was one of the best. It was special that my consultant was there, particularly as I knew Athens was going to be the beginning of the end of my career. I hadn't told anyone, but I knew I wanted to retire after Athens.

Chapter 18

The End of the Road

I was asked to take part in the London Parade of Champions after Athens. At first, I wasn't going to do it. They wanted all the medallists there. Peter Norfolk was out of the country playing a tournament so they wanted me to represent tennis.

Once again the British Paralympic Association and the BBC showed their true colours. The BBC were only interested in certain Olympians, mainly Amir Khan and Kelly Holmes. With the Paralympians, they were interested in Ade, the lad in the wheelchair you see before certain BBC programmes come on. They also focused heavily on Tanni Grey Thompson, which was interesting as she wasn't even at the parade.

What annoyed me was that, before the parade, we were in the hotel and I was talking to a couple of the basketball squad and Leon Taylor, the high diver. The press officer, the one who came up with the *literally a minute* line in Athens, walked by and said 'hello' to everybody, except me.

On the parade bus, we went from Hyde Park to Trafalgar Square. The BBC had a camera on the bus I was on.

I was on the same bus as Amir Khan, a few of the wheelchair basketball players and the Badminton lot. They spoke to the basketball players (who won bronze) and the badminton players (who won silver), but apparently, I wasn't worth an interview. They then left the bus.

Once we got to Trafalgar Square we all got on to the main stage. There were thousands of people crammed in to Trafalgar Square. However, only a few people were interviewed on stage.

Not surprisingly, they were the same people who had been interviewed on the bus and, not surprisingly, they were asked the exact same questions.

Things got worse from there. When it all finished, I had to get back to the hotel from Trafalgar Square. I was told by one of the event organisers that the bus going back to the hotel had no wheelchair access, so I would have to get a taxi!

That cost me over twenty quid.

The main reason for the parade was to support the 'Back London' Olympics bid. They wanted to show they supported the Paralympics as well: the whole thing was a PR exercise. The only positive aspect from a personal point of view was going through a crowd of that size.

THE QUEEN AND HER ASHTRAY

After Athens, the Paralympic team was invited to Buckingham Palace to meet the Queen. The British Tennis Foundation paid for us to stay in a hotel on Kensington High Street. We all got togged up in our suits and went down to the Palace. We went inside and it must have been two hours before the Queen even showed up, by which time I was a bit drunk as there were butlers going round with trays of free ale.

Then, one of my mates rang up and told me to rob something out of the Palace.

Opportunity knocked in the gents. They had set up some wheelchair accessible portacabin toilets inside the Palace itself.

It was quite bizarre. I went in the posh gents, which was full of flowers. There was a painting on the wall and I thought it would look even nicer in my front room, however I would have looked slightly suspicious leaving the front door of the Queen's house with a painting tucked under my arm. I somehow mysteriously acquired an ashtray. A bit disappointing really, because it just looks like a normal ashtray and has nothing on it to show it's from the Palace.

I eventually gave it to someone to sell in a car boot sale.

Then, the Queen came in and spoke to us: 'Oh, hello, and what do you do?'

'I collect ashtrays, love.'

I was surprised at how small she was: Her Majesty would have made an ideal jockey!

I had the impression that when the Queen does stuff like that she is on autopilot, saving all her brain energy. Basically, her eyebrows move and that is about it. When she asked me what I did, I felt like asking her the same question or saying, 'I play tennis and I'm pissed as a fart, fancy a kebab?'

She'd probably seen me with the ashtray on CCTV. Prince Edward then came in and clocked me. I better tell you we had a little history between us.

In Athens, during the doubles semi-final against the Dutch, I was chasing after a ball and wasn't looking where I was going. I reached the ball but crashed head first into the fence. Prince Edward and Sue Wolstenholme were sat a few feet away.

As I hit the fence I shouted out, 'Mark, you fucking spastic!'

I looked up and the Prince was laughing. He left three-quarters through the match as he had other matches to see, but he phoned up later to see how we had got on. The next day, he came down to the village and asked if he could speak to me, but I was having physio at the time so I couldn't.

Now, at Buckingham Palace, Edward came over and said, 'Ah Mark, you're the chap who I saw in the tennis match, and what was it you said?'

Afterwards, we all went to the Sports Café in London and I drank even more. It was like a scrapyard, there were about a hundred wheelchairs in there. I was just looking outside expecting to see the big yellow bus. There's nothing funnier – or should that be horrific? – than seeing eight or nine wheelchairs on the dance floor. CARNAGE!

I just kept thinking 'don't do this to me'.

But it was a good experience on the whole. I've done a few of those kinds of gigs. The Lawn Tennis Association once asked me to go down to London with other sports personalities before an election. I went down with John Crowther, the then boss of the Association. I couldn't believe it when he said to me he was getting slaughtered.

Tony Blair came over to us. I think he knew John, who introduced me. All of a sudden Blair grabbed my shoulders and said, 'Ooh my, you've got big shoulders, haven't you?'

I thought AYE AYE!!

I didn't know what was going on. He asked me what I did so I told him and then he went.

Er, bye then!

I only stayed half an hour. I had to drive back to St Helens, and stay sober! At these events, you can tell who is genuinely interested in you and who isn't.

There are some people, though, who I'd love to sit down with on a one on one basis and ask them a few questions – sportsmen, politicians mainly. There are a few of them who I look at and consider it a burning injustice that they are making more money than me!

Bitter?

Absolutely!

I just want to know how they do it – that's all.

Many footballers aren't hard and spend more money getting their hair done than a girl. Yet they make thousands of pounds a week. And the times they kick wide or over the bar.

The WAGS – I just feel like telling them to get a job in a supermarket or fast food outlet instead of sponging off very rich footballers.

Do you think if footballers were brickies and they got caught shagging grannies, their girlfriends would still be with them?

Thought not.

Good grief. I'd love to bottle how some of these people have made money.

Anyway back to Planet Earth.

I only did two tournaments after Athens, one being the Nottingham indoor, which I won. My contract ran until April 2005 and I wasn't intending to sign for another year. The sooner I was out of it the better, as far as I was concerned.

We were all called to a meeting of wheelchair tennis players in Birmingham to talk about plans for the future. Everybody who was getting some kind of funding was there. A woman from UK Sports turned up to give a talk about lottery funding. About eight players received lottery funding at that point, including myself. We were told that due to a drop in lottery ticket sales, funding was to be reduced. They added that they wanted more medals in Beijing and had come up with a strategy to work out how sports were allocated their funding. In each sport, for every gold medal you had won in Athens, you would receive two spots for lottery funding. For every silver and bronze you won, you would get one spot.

Basically, they were saying they were only keeping three tennis players on lottery funding. Nobody saw this coming, and everyone who had been relying on that money began to panic.

I saw a hole in their strategy – they were cutting spots off the lottery funding, yet expected more medals in Beijing.

Brilliant!

I didn't think I would be one of the three to receive funding even if I was going to carry on. I went over to Sue Wolstenholme and told her that I thought the whole thing was bang out of order. She said that I had intimated that I'd be retiring after Athens anyway. She mentioned my shoulder problems and asked if I could get a letter from my consultant to clarify my condition. It seemed to me like she was looking for a reason to get rid of me but, what she didn't know, was I had already jumped.

I got a letter from Mr Soni in which he confirmed the condition of my shoulder. I had to do this because when you retire through injury your funding goes on for an extra three months, so I sent a copy to Sue along with my resignation letter. That was it for me.

The end of the road.

My last official tournament was the final of the Nationals in 2005. I won the semi-final and straight afterwards the drugs tester came to me and said I'd been selected to do a test. I told them that I was retiring the day after and questioned the wisdom of them testing me. I asked what would they do if they found anything in my system. Ban me? They told me that rules were rules. It was madness really, especially considering each test cost between £200 and £300. They asked me if I had any ID on me, I didn't, so they had to get the tournament director to verify that I was in fact Mark Eccleston. I jokingly gave them the old 'don't you know who I am?' line to which he replied 'no'.

The cheek.

I was in there for about an hour because I couldn't 'go'. This was down to the fact that I'd had to go to the toilet during the game.

The night before the final I got drunk, the reason being because by this time it was common knowledge that I was calling it a day after the Nationals, yet I didn't get a word said about me at the tournament dinner. Other retirees were mentioned, good players, but ones who hadn't achieved anywhere near as much as I had. The only time my name came up was when Pete Norfolk went up to receive his Player of the Year award and they said that he won a silver medal partnering me in Athens.

I found this slightly insulting – although not surprising.

I was laughing because I knew it was coming, but people around me told me that they thought it was out of order.

I got slaughtered at the dinner and then played the final next day. Pete Norfolk beat me easily. It was funny really. He was the last person to beat me and sent me into retirement with a hammering. But, what he doesn't know is, that I was still inebriated from the night before.

Earlier in the week I had said that, if required, I would help the Great Britain team at the World Team Cup if they were struggling. Due to what happened at the dinner, my heart just wasn't in it anymore, and so I officially retired from tennis in April 2005.

MY RECORD

I have represented Great Britain at two Paralympic games in two different sports.

I have played sport at performance level since I was eleven, and I have to say that I prefer team sports to individual sports any day. You can probably tell by reading this book that I enjoyed playing tennis but didn't really enjoy the tennis environment – nowhere near as much as I enjoyed the rugby one. This was mainly down to the fact that there are more muppets in tennis than there are in rugby.

A perfect example of this is a wheelchair tennis player who said he would rather be in a wheelchair and be a millionaire, than be on his feet!

I rest my case.

I think that is pathetic. I would rather be on my feet, skint and selling the *Big Issue* than be in a wheelchair, loaded and World No 1.

The mindset of a team player and an individual player are worlds apart.

In some situations, it's quite disturbing the lengths that some people will go to win in an individual sport. For example, at one tennis tournament, a player was playing a match in extremely hot conditions. One of his entourage was asked to get some ice for the opponent. They were given an ice vest to pass it on but they never did. After the match, the person that the ice vest had been intended for fell extremely ill. Apparently, so I was told, an investigation was conducted but, as far as I'm aware, no action was taken. This absolutely horrified me.

During my appraisal with the British Tennis Foundation at the end of 2004, I made them aware of my knowledge of the incident. You should have seen their faces.

Priceless!!

Nothing like this ever happened in rugby!

Don't get me wrong; wheelchair sport has given me a great life.

I have travelled the world and I have no regrets. Idiots exist in all walks of life and the fact that politics exist in wheelchair sport can be taken as a positive, as it means it's getting more professional. However, I have met some idiots in all walks of life and disability sport is no different.

Chapter 19

Psychology – Eccy Style

My competitive career had to end at some point. I didn't want to damage my shoulder any further and, as I have mentioned, my career was all about setting goals. I had achieved the goals I'd set myself so I no longer felt motivated to carry on.

There were also a number of people I preferred not to deal with again.

I never ever said I wanted to win Paralympic Gold. I always said I wanted a Paralympic medal. Granted, I would rather it was gold.

I also wanted to be World No 1 and World Champion. So I attained all three of my goals. The effort and commitment required to participate in Beijing in 2008 was beyond what I felt I was capable of. At Athens I realised that I would not be able to perform to the levels I wanted to any longer; mentally and physically, it would be too much for me. Being in a chair for twenty years catches up with you; your shoulders are not designed to take the strains and stresses that mine have been put under. I wouldn't have been able to do myself justice in Beijing and I have always believed that if you're going to do a job, you should do it properly.

Getting into coaching seemed a natural progression. I had learned a lot over the years and felt I could pass some of that knowledge on. I also had some sense of history.

In 1984–85, I was 14 years old and Australian legend Mal Meninga signed for Saints. That was a huge boost for the club and the town. I was a ball boy for Saints at the time. After the match, you'd go up to the players' lounge and mix with them, and the traditional rugby league delicacy of pie and peas would be on offer.

Meninga came to our school one day and watched us practice. He noticed that Moff and me were the main men and came over to talk to us.

We started discussing training and he said that he couldn't believe how many six-mile runs he had to go on at the Saints. He said he never went on six-mile runs during a game so couldn't understand why he had to do it in training. It was then that I realised Australian training was all games based, and that that was one of the reasons why we were so far behind them.

This lesson came back to me much later in my tennis career. When I changed coaches to work with Phil Leighton, he made me do a lot of games-based drills, which I had never done in tennis training before. I had been able to get to No 3 in the world, but just couldn't make the final step to No 1, mainly because what I was doing in practice did not reflect what I would have to do in competitive play. Phil would make me do things exactly like I would in a game. I was a bit annoyed with myself that it had taken someone else to tell me why I wasn't No 1 in the world, especially considering Meninga had already hinted at it in 1984.

Now I am coaching, I make sure my training style is games-based.

I had done a bit of coaching previously in schools and a little with Phil. If you play your cards right and know what you're doing, you can become quite successful. Put it this way: you never see a good tennis coach with a broken alarm clock or a bad car.

Going into schools is enjoyable too. Like anything though, you need the qualifications and certificates to prove you can do it. I decided to do my coaching qualification so I could coach professionally. My course was going to be paid for by the Lawn Tennis Association so I had nothing to lose. I saw that it would give me more clout and make me legit.

The course involved a lot of time-consuming writing but it wasn't difficult. There are three levels and you can't progress until you have completed the level before. For what I want to do, maybe somewhere down the line I will need level 2. There is no point me doing a level 3 because that is a performance level which allows you to coach the likes of Tim Henman and Andy Murray. Mentally I could help them in telling them how to win a match, but, physically, I wouldn't be capable of hitting with them due to the level of my injury.

Going on the course was both eye-opening and saddening. It made me realise why British tennis is in the sorry state it currently finds itself in. My rule is simple; I judge coaches on whether I would want to be coached by them or whether I would send my kids to be coached by them. Half the people on my course should never have got anywhere near a tennis centre but some passed. I suppose it's all about quotas these days.

I have to say that I didn't learn much more than I already knew – but now I am certified to coach. I am coaching individual wheelchair tennis players, as well as going into schools, because it's a specialist sport that requires specialist coaches. I keep going back to it: some of the coaches who are involved in wheelchair tennis in this country are not of the standard the sport requires or deserves. In my opinion at least.

It annoys me so much, because there are good players out there, good players who came through the ranks with me, who have left the sport because of the way they were treated.

I think that's terrible.

I've seen players who are on the programme, getting funding and competing for Great Britain spots, who would be beaten convincingly by some of the people I have seen leave the sport.

The development side of the British Tennis Federation has done well but the performance side don't always get it right. Let me give an example. In December 2006, the Cliff Richard Tennis Foundation and asked me if I would like to attend the Cliff Richard Classic Tennis event and give a demonstration of wheelchair tennis.

Of course, I accepted the offer. I took along Carl Hird, a player

I was training with and who I now coach. We went down to Birmingham on the Saturday morning. I was under the impression that we were just going to do a wheelchair tennis demo. When we got there, they asked us to do a demonstration, but that wasn't all. Then we would be split up with one of us going on Coronation Street star Bradley Walsh's side and the other joining Cliff's team. We went into the VIP lounge where we met all the celebrities. We did our demo in front of a packed house of 10,000. Then we played mixed doubles with Virginia Wade and Annabel Croft. We went to the party afterwards and only got home at 3 a.m. the next morning. I asked one of the organisers why they didn't contact the British Tennis Federation to arrange some players to attend the event.

They said they had but were told no one was available.

I found that a bit strange because the event was shown on TV on Christmas Day. What better time to give the sport some free exposure!

You know you've made it if you're on TV on Christmas day!

Sometimes you go to events and feel you are only there as a token gesture. The Cliff Richard Tennis Classic was different because we were made to feel an important part of the event. It was very enjoyable day and all those involved were superb with us. They were genuinely interested in knowing more about Wheelchair Tennis.

I was on Cliff's team and if someone who was sat next to me got up to play, he would come over and have a chat with me. Other players included GMTV's Penny Smith, Angus Deayton, Jasper Carrott and Joe Pasquale.

Sir Cliff Richard

With the Cliff Richard Foundation now providing opportunities for children with disabilities to play tennis, it was fantastic that Mark could join us at the Tennis Classic. His achievements are truly inspirational and his participation in the Tennis Classic helped to make the day a huge success.

I have no idea why the British Tennis Federation didn't send a couple of players to the event. An opportunity was there to appear on Sky Sports on Christmas Day and it wasn't taken, but I certainly wasn't going to turn that chance down.

BECOMING COACH

If you're the first tetraplegic to become a qualified tennis coach in the world and your governing body doesn't send you a letter congratulating you, something's amiss. I have been asked by a number of people if I think it's personal. I would like to think not.

I believe it will come to the point, though, where certain people would rather have me on side than not, because they will eventually dispense with their arrogance and realise I know a lot more than they do.

I've been there and done it.

I know what it takes to be World No 1 and, more mundanely, I know how tournaments and travel arrangements work; I know the wheelchair sports scene inside out. I'm not coaching to boost my ego; I'm doing it because I feel it would be such a waste not to pass on what I've learned.

If anyone I coach were to get to World No 1 or win a tournament, I won't be jumping in to all the photos saying, 'Look at me, I'm the coach', like some I could mention. I don't want any of that. I will stay in the background and I won't be doing interviews as it's not my achievement. It will be the player's achievement. I will have just helped them along the way.

I feel that I have got a lot to offer players. Parts of coaching sometimes do make you think 'why am I bothering?' But I love the actual on-court coaching. The off-court politics and some of the clowns involved are a pain. Unfortunately, they are part and parcel of any sport.

A big thing in my coaching is that I've learnt from the best. The most successful wheelchair rugby coach is Terry Vinyard, who I played under at Tampa.

The best coach I ever worked with, full stop, who understood me, knew what made me tick, and knew how to get the best out of me, is Brian Worrall.

The best wheelchair tennis coach I've ever seen is Jason Harnett.

And then there's Craig and Phil whose guidance and input contributed significantly to making me being the best quad tennis player in the world.

I have picked things up from all of them, and I'd be a fool not to tap into all of those resources. One of my great sources of strength as a coach is my ability to man-manage; I know how to deal with people as individuals. A lot of coaches treat people as a group or exactly the same. That's not the way it should be done. Players are individuals. Some people need an arm round them and need to be told they are a great player. Others just need a kick up the arse, with the words 'GET ON WITH IT' ringing and stinging in their ears.

It would be very interesting to coach another Mark Eccleston.

I'd trust him and probably do it more or less the same way Brian Worrall did. I'd say if he let me down, we'd be finished, but I'd know he wouldn't let me down. Every now and then I'd give him a bit of a bollocking for messing around, because champions tend to be the sort who occasionally do. I'd also boost his confidence at times. Believe it or not, there were times when I would doubt myself and Brian would tell me what a good player I was. I sometimes needed that during my rugby career because, if we'd lose heavily as a team, I would blame myself, as I was the main man on the team and captain. Brian would always know what to say on these occasions to wallop my confidence back up.

I've also coached wheelchair rugby. I coached Southport while playing for them when we won the national championships. I got them training properly as, previously, training would just be a messing around session. I insisted we discuss tactics and set pieces – and we won nationals. I've been asked about coaching wheelchair rugby again. Part of me feels that when I left rugby for tennis I left rugby behind for good.

Would I go back? A few questions have been asked as to

whether I might be interested in being involved again. I have to admit I have thought about it because I am still a team sports person at heart.

Maybe I might get involved eventually in some way. I wouldn't be able to put everything into wheelchair rugby though, as I have other things going on now.

The team 'thing' shines through with my tennis coaching, as I make all my players train together. In the past, certain players just wanted to do things as individuals. As a coach, I'm not having that. There have been players involved in the Great Britain set-up in the past who have said they would not come down to a training session as there was no one good enough to hit with them, and they have got away with that. Sorry, but if you're a good coach you can design a drill which will benefit every player. The players I am coaching at the moment all have to hit with each other. For one thing, there's no point in hitting against the same person all the time. I go through the drills and tactics with them but, when it comes to match play, there's no point. I am a left-hander so when you play against a right-hander, you won't be used to it. You need to play against people with different styles.

Anthony Cotterill, *Great Britain wheelchair tennis player*

I met Mark whilst I was in hospital. I did a tennis beginner's camp in Nottingham and met Mark there. I started to go across to the tennis centre where Mark trained. As he got more into the coaching, I wanted him as a coach, as he has been there, done that. Player wise, he knows a lot more about a disability sport than an able bodied coach.

He's hard as a coach. Hard, but fair. If you're not playing well you'll get a bollocking, which is how it should be – and how I like it. On the other hand, he's quick to praise you.

He's had a massive impact on my career. Up until very recently, I was probably lacking a bit of confidence. Mark has always said to me that one day it will all come together for me and that he has belief in me. Now it is all coming together and I'm starting to believe in myself. I've just won a title in Sunderland, all the hard work is starting to pay off. Everything he has ever said has been right, he knows how to play the sport; the proof is in the pudding.

Jamie Burdekin, *Great Britain wheelchair tennis player*

I asked Mark to be my coach because of what he's done in his past. I wanted to learn from the best. I was introduced to the game just as he was finishing off. When he was at his best he was unbeatable. His mind games worked; psychologically he had a lot of players beat before he went on court. You can only learn off that.

He's brilliant as a coach, you go on court and you're not his mate anymore; he's hard. He says what he thinks – training has a disciplined approach – and he pushes you. I'd sooner have it like that. There's no messing around; you do what he says and get the job done. You always know where you stand with him.

He's a good lad and we have a good laugh off the court. What you see is what you get with Mark. We've been everywhere together and had a ball, like the time in our hotel Australia when we had front row seats at a Valentine's Night Sex show!

As for something not so nice I'd like to say about him, his shit stinks! No, just joking, he's a great man to work with.

If you ever need anything off him he's there for you, apart from being stingy with his money! He's a cracking lad and he has definitely helped develop my career. He's a huge part in how far I've come over the last few years.

The British Tennis Foundation, over the years, has had control of wheelchair tennis in Great Britain. The development side of the foundation, led by Lynn Parker, has done a fantastic job in promoting the sport and organising and running camps and tournaments. Unfortunately, the same cannot be said for the performance side. Britain is probably the best funded wheelchair tennis country so why aren't we the most successful? Pete Norfolk and I were both successful in spite of the perfomance side, not because of it. The performance side of wheelchair tennis in Britain has gone backwards over the last few years and I'm afraid I blame some of the coaches in charge. Let me give you an example. The men's team that GB took to the World Team Cup in 2006 to Brazil and Sweden in 2007 were the weakest I have ever seen; in fact, in 2006 the men's team got relegated into World Group 2 after losing to Thailand! I'm sorry, no offence to Thailand, but that is embarrassing. The Quad team that won the World Team Cup in 2001 and 2002 would have beaten them and that should never be the case.

I went on a tennis camp once and saw coaches who shouldn't even be on a tennis court, and yet they had the job of guiding the destiny of some of our brightest talent. I was excited to see how good some of the UK players were. Within five years we should be able to dominate wheelchair tennis. But there's an 'if' which stops me getting too optimistic; I'm afraid our best talent is in the hands of some people who don't know their arse from their elbow.

I used to get frustrated when coaches, who I felt were not up to the level I demanded, would come over and give me advice. If I'm getting beaten by people I shouldn't be losing to, or my standards are slipping, fine, come and tell me. However, I was World No 1, winning tournaments all over the world so, excuse cocky old Mark, I don't see why I should listen to people who know as much about wheelchair tennis as I do about splitting the atom!

I saw one coach, saying to the players, 'So and so plays a shot like this', when I knew full well that so and so didn't. This coach really doesn't understand how you have to play if you are in a wheelchair; the way he was coaching these players could lead to them being injured within a year.

The discipline you need to reach and keep a competitive standard is tough. Training in the UK when, on a winter's morning, you have to get up in the dark and work in the cold can be trying.

Having said that, I have no sympathy with athletes who say that the training conditions in the UK, as compared to Australia or the USA, are a reason why we don't get the success. That's a cop-out, an excuse. If you're saying that type of thing you shouldn't be competing in the first place. It's a loser's mentality. Realistically, most top British sports people will do warm weather training anyway.

The big problem with sport in this country is bad coaches.

I've done my coaching qualification now and I want to help nurture talent, not set it back. I remember when I needed a hitting partner and the able-bodied coaches I was working with couldn't sustain more than a four shot rally with me, so what were they doing there in the first place?

Britain needs someone to coach the coaches, I'd say.

THE PSYCHOLOGY OF CROWDS

Crowd reaction is an interesting subject. I've played in a lot of matches where the crowd has been negative towards me. I'm one of those people who thrives on hostility, it spurs me on. I'm confrontational: if someone wants to argue with me, I'm always happy to oblige. It's a stimulant. A lot of other people find arguing too much for them to deal with.

When I was playing rugby for Great Britain and we'd head over to the US and Canada, the crowd broke a few British players. You see it in tennis players, too. Some players don't like the crowd getting involved.

But I love it. Don't get me wrong; there have been occasions when I've had the crowd with me. I remember the doubles semi-final against Holland in Athens. It was a predominantly British crowd. A section in the corner was supporting Holland and I've got to say the Dutch supporters were fantastic. They made a lot of noise and they all wore orange. The British supporters got behind us that day. When they do that, it gives you a lift and increases your adrenaline. Your body responds as you feel them rooting for you. Some players like the positive crowds, but can't handle the negative ones. I'm equally at home with both. I'm not slagging people off who can't handle an opposition crowd because it is intimidating and very personal with tennis. In rugby you're out there as part of a team. In tennis, it's just you.

Some of the stuff I've had said to me is unbelievable. You can usually judge if it's somebody doing it just because they think it's clever. I always react by laughing it off and asking them how many world titles they've won. That soon shuts them up.

The Americans, with Jason in charge, had the attitude that they would not stoop down to that level and they did not, but I will go head to head with anyone in terms of 'sledging' as the Aussies call it. I'm not saying I'll win every time, but I'll give it a good go. People like Jason and Pete Norfolk wouldn't get involved and would stay quiet.

I also got slagged off a lot by the authorities because of my behaviour. What they didn't realise was that a part of my success was due to my behaviour. Ninety per cent of the time I was doing it to unsettle my opponent. The Aussies have done it for years – and brilliantly in the Ashes in 2006. I was never nasty, though, and I never did anything that was against the rules.

I was brought up to believe that if someone has a go at you, you have a go back. You look after yourself. There is no difference between being bullied on a school playground and some of the abuse I got in a sporting arena. The Israelis were the masters of this style of play, and they could be sly. Either way, I can't stand bullies and I will take them on any day.

Mental images helped me. With certain players I always had a swan in mind. Quiet and calm on the surface, but paddling like mad underneath. I don't think a number of top players liked playing me; I think they thought I was nuts.

I was the McEnroe of wheelchair tennis. People who aren't educated, or haven't a clue what they are talking about, thought McEnroe was a troublemaker, but he wasn't. Look at the success he achieved. Most of what he did, he meant to do. His arguments with the umpires, and everything else he did, disrupted the momentum of his opponents. In any sport, momentum is king. When you're on top, you're on top. Anyone with any brains, who is losing, will do something to try and shift the momentum.

Technically, I wasn't the best player in the world. I wasn't the fastest player in the world. I wasn't the strongest player in the world. If you tick all these boxes I wasn't top in any of them, except, maybe, for the best forehand.

However, psychologically I was best by far. My mental attitude compensated – and more than – for the deficiencies in my game.

I began to tap into psychology with Dr Clive Glass who, like Mr Soni, first saw me soon after my accident.

Dr Clive Glass – *clinical psychologist*

Mark approached me in May 1996 and we began to discuss how he might develop his game. At that time there was little consideration in wheelchair tennis circuit of the importance of psychological preparation, and it would be fair to say that Mark realised this well before the majority of his competitors. He would visit the Centre at the end of the clinical day and we began discussing how he might match his technical understanding of the game and his opponents' strengths and weaknesses with how he might approach and play his games.

We did two main things together. I showed him how to visualise shots and minimise the risk of faults by imagining that the area to attack was a much larger area than he at first identified. I also taught him how to relax and stay focused during points and rest breaks. He also was looking to find a system to keep himself cool in hot weather.

He managed to win a number of tournaments and established himself at Number 1 in the World Rankings. He then experienced a problem with his shoulder. As he had to rest and not compete, with the possibility he might not be able to play again, he required considerably more support at this time. He also had to cope with the drop in world ranking position as others, who he knew he was capable of beating, began to overtake him. As his injury settled, he began tournament tennis again. But he started losing games and matches to people he felt he should beat.

By getting him to concentrate on the positive points in games and identify the reasons why shots went wrong, slowly he began to re-establish his confidence. We played to his strengths, rather than his weaknesses, and developed game plans to unsettle his opponents; for example, devising strategies to slow down those who favoured quick games, and to flip the situation on players who used the break rules to their advantage. At the international level, the technical level of competitors is always likely to be relatively equal – on any day any one of half a dozen people might win the competition. What matters is the approach taken to the game and the ability to maintain a competitive advantage.

Had Mark believed the title was his by right, he would have failed. He was always able to maintain a balance between confidence and a healthy respect for his opponents. That confidence is an attribute which I believe was within him before his injury – I am sure his family will testify to his independence and abilities – but after the experience of the injury, once he had accommodated what he could do (and found difficulty with) physically, any other challenge became much simpler. He has said, in many ways over the years, that if he could get his head around his injuries, he could get his head around anything, including being a world champion. I do not say being able to deal with being a world champion lightly – don't forget that once you are there you have to work doubly hard to stay there – for the points system means, essentially, that you have to reach the final or win the majority of tournaments you enter. You also have to deal with the likelihood of not staying there, and Mark accomplished this well.

If you get involved with tennis coaching you will be told to read *Winning Ugly* by Brad Gilbert, who now coaches Andy Murray. His book does what it says on the tin, so to speak. It tells you how to win ugly. Gilbert was no great shakes as a player. Technically, he wasn't the best but he beat a lot of the top players during his career. Psychologically, he had it.

I believe that Roger Federer is the best tennis player of all time. Without a doubt, he will break every record. As a junior, you would never have thought it, then someone got hold of him and taught him how to win. It was the same with Gilbert; he learnt how to beat someone with his mind. In any sport, *by and large*, you'll win more than you lose if you're tough mentally.

There are sayings that, when it came to big tournaments, I used to have written down. One of the books I took a lot from was *What It Takes to be Number One* by the renowned American Football coach, Vince Lombardi.

Some of his points are really wise.

'While statistics are interesting they're all in the past' – if I'm playing someone who has beaten me ten times in the past, it's not a great statistic but I'm not playing them ten times today. It's only the present match that matters. At some point down the line, I will beat them, as I managed to do with Draney. I did not beat him for years, but I worked hard and eventually got my rewards.

'Study the past, live in the present' – you just have to learn from your mistakes you make and rectify them now.

'Your focus is not on what is actually happening to you but on what you think is happening to you. Over time, this self talk can relate into belief, a positive or negative opinion of yourself and your circumstances, it is this internal opinion, positive or negative that determines your thoughts, actions, habits and ultimately your character.'

You're playing a match and you hit a couple of bad shots, and all of a sudden you start thinking you are rubbish. If you think that often enough, it becomes a self-fulfilling prophecy and your game will collapse.

All you've done, however, is play two bad shots out of God knows how many, so you're not really playing badly at all. Get a grip. Perception becomes reality. If you think something enough then it's going to happen that way.

Lombardi was light years ahead of his time.

'Without turmoil, there's no growth. Without turmoil, there's no strength and ultimately no improvement.'

You have to learn to enjoy the tough days and meet them head on. If you do, the good days will arrive and when they do they will taste so much sweeter.

'Cream always rises to the top.'

'Form is temporary, class is permanent.'

If you are good at something and you go through a bad patch, you need to work harder and, if you do, it will all come good again.

These sayings all relate to the same thing. If everything is rosy for you, what have you got to look forward to and get excited about?

If you have a bad day at the office, it's almost as good as having a great day. This is because you go away hating the feeling of under-performing. That's why in sport, someone will take a hammering and, very often, they will go on and win their next game. They remember the pain of defeat all too clearly, and don't want to experience it again. You have to go through the rough days if you want to be successful – not just in sport, but in life as well.

Flying home from America with my right arm dangling lifelessly was a rough day. Being told that would be about it for my career was a terrible moment. Still, I overcame these traumas in the end.

My favourite saying is *'How a person masters his fate is more important than what that fate is.'*

It is all about how you react to adversity. If you react positively you will go on to be more successful than if you react negatively.

The big thing is that, until the day you die, you should always have your eyes and ears open ready to learn something. I remember key things I am told. A lot of people underestimate the mental side of sport; they think just because they can move fast or have the physical attributes, then it's enough. They couldn't be more wrong.

The perfect example of maybe not being the most gifted participant in a sporting contest, but being the most mentally strong and never giving in was the 2005 Champions League final between my beloved Liverpool and AC Milan, a match that will never be forgotten.

Liverpool were 3–0 down at half time. The Liverpool coach Rafa Benitez told his players in the interval that they played for Liverpool, and that if they didn't go out in the second half and play their best, they didn't deserve to wear the Liverpool shirt. Rafa told them to think of all the fans. He put it into their head that they still had a chance.

The rest is history.

Brian Clough, one of the greatest football managers ever, came out with a great quote:

'*It only takes a second to score a goal.*'

If you work on that theory, Liverpool had to find three goal-scoring seconds in 45 minutes of football. You've got a lot of time, in fact, when you look at it like that.

The difference between Liverpool and Milan was that Milan started getting nervy as soon as Liverpool scored their first goal. The second goal had Milan's sphincter twitching like a bunny rabbit's nose and floored them completely. Mentally they didn't have the nous to do something that would change the momentum that had obviously shifted Liverpool's way.

That's where I can help when coaching because, mentally, I was always very strong. It didn't just come to me. I studied it. I have read hundreds of books – particularly autobiographies of people I looked up to and respected, such as the basket ball player, Michael Jordan, and the cyclist, Lance Armstrong. His book is good even if at some stages it is quite corny.

Australian Rugby League player Ian Robert's book is also very good. He was the first high profile rugby league player to come out as a homosexual. He did it even though he knew he would be in for a very hard time. He had to deal with all the abuse and negativity thrown his way. Not only did he do that but he went on to become one of the top forwards of his generation.

I'll never say I have a hero; I have people I respect and admire. I try and get as much information out of them as possible. It applies to all aspects of life, not just sport. If you have a negative attitude, then you're not going to achieve much. Reading how stars psyched themselves up to achieve, studying their sayings, helps me immensely.

I want to read about stuff that has actually happened, true stories. I also like to read about murders and serial killers for some reason.

When I went to Atlanta in 1996, I had a few sayings stuck up on my bedroom wall. People who saw it either asked what it was all about or they took the piss.

I had the last laugh because I came away with a certificate

confirming I was the outstanding British wheelchair rugby player at the Paralympics. There are a lot of people in life who don't tap into the mental side of things as much as they should. Mental and physical strength work in tandem.

SPORT IS GOOD FOR YOU

A study in Canada found that physical activity in a person with a spinal cord injury reduces the time spent in hospital by 6 to 8 eight weeks. That's a long time. I have never suffered all the illnesses and ailments commonly associated with my injury, such as kidney infections, bladder infections, chest infections, pressure sores, and, touch wood, I never will. I put it down to the fact that I'm so active.

Again, this translates to all walks of life. If you're active you're going to reduce the chances of getting ill. Your immune system strengthens and it makes you more alert mentally. If you go out for a walk or go to the gym, it has positive benefits. If you take up sport professionally there are financial benefits too as well as, if you're lucky, getting to see the world. For every level, from somebody taking their dog for a walk to somebody going to the Paralympics, there are benefits to an active lifestyle. I really believe more could be done to promote this.

If you go to Australia, go past any park and you will see people playing rugby league, cricket, throwing Frisbees and so on. They say the climate is a major influence on maintaining an active lifestyle but you also see a lot of TV adverts in Australia promoting health. If something is put in your head often enough you will do it without thinking. It's 'muscle memory'. As a tennis player, you do something over and over again, and eventually there is joy in repetition because, when you come to a match, you do it automatically. It's the same with lifestyle. How many fat people do you see on TV in the UK? They come on TV moaning that they have an illness or they have a disease. With some people that may very well be the case, but with others it's habit and weakness; they open the fridge, they eat rubbish.

CONFIDENCE IS NOT ARROGANCE

OK, for those that don't know, let's sort out the difference between arrogance and confidence. The problem I have with a lot of people – and it is usually people who haven't achieved much in their life or think they are lot better than they actually are – is that they mistake confidence for arrogance.

A lot of people have called me arrogant. I'm not arrogant. I have never said that I'm going to do something that I'm not capable of doing. I'm confident, because everything I've I said I was going to do, I have done. There have been occasions when I have gone on to remind those who doubted me, but they had it coming.

St Helens rugby legend, Alex Murphy, gives the best definition: 'People mistake confidence for arrogance. With me, it's not arrogance because I can do it.'

My view is this: with arrogance, you think you can do it. With confidence, you can do it.

With arrogance, you don't listen to other people. With confidence, you are constantly listening.

Whenever Phil Leighton told me to do something, I did it. Whenever Jason spoke to me, I took heed. Whenever Brian Worrall offered advice after he had bollocked me in Dallas, I acted upon it. If you're arrogant, you won't listen because you think you don't need to. Any great athlete will tell you that, somewhere down the line, there was a mentor who they viewed as a God and always heeded religiously. Every older Liverpool player who is interviewed would mention Bill Shankly. The Liverpool players from the next era would mention Bob Paisley.

I imagine I annoyed some of my coaches because I would always be asking them questions, trying to become a better player. When I was in the States, I would hound Terry Vinyard. Tactically, he was light years ahead of everyone else. When I was flying to tournaments with Tampa, I would always try and make sure I was sat next to Terry. And I could see the poor bloke rolling his eyes as I peppered him with questions.

If someone accuses of me being arrogant these days, I just say, 'Read the CV.'

They're facts.

That's the way my mum and dad brought me up – if you're going to do something, do it properly. I think with careers, maybe the decision is made for you. Sometimes it was a disadvantage being the youngest in the family, and sometimes it was a motivation, wanting to better what my brothers had done. I have had a successful sporting career because my older brothers were good at sport. If they had been excellent gardeners, I would probably have gone into flower arranging.

You've just got to go out there and do it. Some people can, some people can't. It's the ones who can't, or don't want to enough, who label you arrogant.

Chapter 20

If I May Say a Few Final Words...

In 2003 I told Mark Bullock, the International Tennis Federation Wheelchair Development Officer, that I would always be happy to help with their work. The Federation have a silver fund than runs in conjunction with the Johann Cruyff foundation. They go to countries that haven't got wheelchair tennis programmes and help get them started by running coaching clinics.

Mark Bullock said he might well take me up on my offer as, no matter where he travelled, be it Colombia or Peru, there were a lot of quads.

I got an e-mail from Mark in May 2005 saying he was doing a trip to Russia at the invitation of the British Council and would I be interested in coming with him? I said I would be more than happy to help. I flew out to Ekaterinburg, which is in the Ural region. The city is named after Catherine of all the Russias who reigned from when she was seventeen and was possibly the randiest of all royals. According to rumours she even got jiggy with a horse! A thoroughbred, I expect.

But the city named in her honour is a dump!

To be serious, there are people with disabilities there who don't even get out of the house. We stayed in the only five-star hotel, though it would struggle to get a three-star rating in the UK. Everywhere is dusty all day, as the local economy is based on mining minerals. The sky is hazy, and you can feel the dust in your chest.

When we went to the tennis centre, there were ten steps leading up to it – ten of the steepest steps you can imagine. I had to be carried up in my chair. The next day, they had put two planks of wood up as a kind of ramp so that chairs could be wheeled up even in a perilous fashion. To be honest, the Russian ramp was more dangerous than the steps, but they were trying.

We did a demonstration for them. As I was talking to a few of them it became clear that they had nothing. They couldn't get out of their houses because they couldn't afford cars and public transport wasn't wheelchair accessible. Looking round the streets was just like watching a 1960s movie with clapped-out old buses struggling down the road. Every now and then a BMW X5 would go by, but it was a burst of sun on a grey day. Apparently Ekaterinaburg is the main city where drugs come into Russia, as it is right on the border with Asia.

Mark and I went from the hotel to the British Council offices, a distance of a quarter mile. It took us 45 minutes with me being in a chair. There were massive holes on the paths and in the road, and the kerbs were about 3 feet high. People were staring at me as if I had three heads; the residents of Ekaterinburg had obviously not seen many people in wheelchairs before.

We were there to show the people how to play tennis but it soon got into how we were going to help them medically.

One young girl said to me, 'Do you know anyone in London that can cure me?'

Some of them hadn't even got to grips with personal hygiene. It was a real eye opener, but I'm glad I went. One guy who had had his accident whilst serving in the Russian Army received the grand sum of 60 US dollars a month. The government ran a scheme where they paid 40% towards a car if you found the other 60% but, of course, he couldn't afford it. He couldn't go out anywhere.

We took them to a posh restaurant that had a ramp and accessible toilets. We went there for an awards night. You could see they were in awe of their surroundings. When we laid food on for them at the tennis centre, you could see them putting some of it in their bags to take home. The next night, we took them to a bowling alley. We managed to get hold of the only two wheelchair accessible minibuses in the city to take them there. The British Council paid for all of this. In the UK, we would classify the bowling alley as a dump, yet they were all saying, 'What an amazing place.'

I would like to go back one day to see if things have improved. The powers that be there were full of promises on how they would get a tennis programme running; I would like to see if those promises have been fulfilled.

It makes you appreciate what we have over here. It's sad to see high-profile Russian billionaires take their money out of the country, especially when you consider the standard of living some people have to endure.

The hotel and airlines didn't have a clue what to do with someone in a wheelchair either.

Coming home was the best bit. We had to fly from Ekaterinburg to Moscow, then on to Frankfurt and, finally, to Manchester. When we got to the airport at Ekaterinaburg, the staff didn't know what to do with me. One official said, 'Come with me', and led me down this corridor to a dark windowless room where a single lamp shone. A woman with a white coat, her hair tied up in an old fashioned bun said, in a frighteningly deep voice, 'You wait here.'

Long pause.

Then, she said, 'Passport, now.'

I was half expecting the woman to start putting on a pair of rubber gloves, but fortunately she never did.

She was filling in forms and making telephone calls and, after a few minutes, the doors behind her swing open and two blokes burst through. They grab me, lift me down the steps and start pushing me over to the plane. I was praying it was the right plane.

I asked Mark what was going on, only to receive the less than reassuring reply; 'I don't know but I'm not liking it'.

Moscow didn't have a clue on how to handle someone in a wheelchair either but, much to my relief, Frankfurt was a lot better. I've never been so glad to see a German in all my life!

Russia was certainly an experience I will never forget, for a number of reasons, and although I am glad I went, I was very happy to get home.

MY LIFE AS A FAN

If you're a true sports fan, whether it be baseball, basketball, snooker, darts, football or rugby, you end up attached to somebody and it's not your decision. With basketball, I would watch the Chicago Bulls at the time of Michael Jordan. I still keep any eye on how they do now. Everybody's got a favourite in every sport.

Supporting Liverpool runs in the family. My mum, dad and brothers all support Liverpool. You are born to support a team. It makes me laugh when you get celebrity fans like David Mellor who grew up a Fulham fan and then switched to Chelsea – to my cynical mind – when they started to get a bit of success.

I use a Liverpool FC season ticket and go to every home game when I'm here.

Rugby League is also in my roots. I'm still a St Helens lad. My mum, dad and my brothers are all Saints fans. My two brothers both played rugby for the town team. So again, the decision was made for me. Technically, I suppose I should support Widnes because that's where I was officially born. Before my accident, I would watch whoever was at home that week, be it Saints or Widnes. But I'll die a Saints fan, as I was born.

I don't think you can remain neutral when watching any sporting occasion – you have to have an emotional tie to the contest. That's human nature. I can put the TV or radio on and two teams I have no affiliation with can be playing and, yet, I will end up leaning towards one side.

If I'm on a long journey I will always listen to sport on the radio especially if they have live commentary on. I don't care who's playing, but as I'm going down the motorway I find myself automatically leaning towards one team. I'm sure a shrink could explain that.

CHAMPION AND AFTER

Other than coaching, the main thing I'm involved in now is speaking in schools and at corporate events. I really enjoy it, although when I first started it frightened me to death.

It all began in 2003, when I had physiotherapy at the English Institute of Sports. They have an athletes' award programme and this gives you around £1000 per year towards something that will help you when your career is over.

I was entitled to the award but wasn't sure what I'd use the money for. I was then told about a 'Speakers boot camp' weekend where a bloke was coming down to talk about public speaking. I thought I'd give it a go. The bloke was Frank Furness, a renowned global speaker.

I was amazed at the money they were saying you could earn. There were about ten of us on the course. We were told that we would have to speak about our lives for five minutes. I was bricking myself. I spoke about the rugby and the tennis. They then give you feedback on what you've said. They were all saying, 'That's unbelievable, you've done so much.' I was quite taken aback.

At the end of the first day, Furness came over to me and said, 'This is for you; you've got to do this. The story you have is one that people will pay to listen to.'

I've done a few functions since then and it's something I'd like to develop further. You can speak to businesses, schools and after dinner events held by various public and private organisations. With businesses, it's mainly at conventions; I did one in 2005 with a big building company. They'd had poor results the year previously and wanted me to talk about how to deal with adversity. You tailor your speech to your audience. I've done a few teachers' conventions and you change it slightly for them. You slip the odd story and joke in. You talk for 45 minutes, answer a few questions and off you go. 45 minutes may seem a long time but to be honest, my real problem is sticking to the time limit.

The first time I spoke in front of those ten people I was very nervous, but now I speak to 500 people without flinching. I want to get into the after dinner circuit because I can cut out the inhibitions then. I can't go into businesses or schools and start talking about strippers or sex in disabled toilets, can I!

Mike, *Mark's brother, agrees*

I would never have dreamt in a month of Sundays that Mark would have the confidence to talk in front of an audience of strangers. I have not seen him in action, but I know from my job what presenting is like. So to go straight in without any experience is something else. Personally, I find all the things that Mark has achieved to be inspiring. He wasn't a child prodigy in anything, didn't have private lessons or the best coaches. Like most of us, he was an 'average' kid growing up in industrial St Helens.

For me, Mark's achievements put many of life's whinges and bitches into perspective. I am so pleased this book has been written – hopefully many people will get the chance to read it and feel inspired and motivated by Mark's story. As a minimum, every school library should have one! He is the best example I know of someone making the best of the attributes that they have, and their personal circumstance. I wish I had all of Mark's qualities (though maybe not some of his opinions!).

If you can speak well, you can have a real impact on someone's life. When someone starts having self-doubt you can pick them up. I've been there; I have needed inspiration and motivation.

Like the times when it was lashing it down with rain and I had to drive to Wirral for a training session in the cold and dark, knowing I was only going to get back when it was dark. I didn't want to do it. I needed someone to get behind me and encourage me.

Like the times when I was injured and I started doubting my own ability, I needed some one there to pick me up.

I am now giving the same encouragement in both my coaching and speaking and I receive letters back thanking me. They love it, and so do I.

There is a scheme called 'sporting champions' run by Sport England. They have seven or eight elite athletes in each region and you go into schools and talk to the kids or do a coaching session. The good thing about kids is they will tell it like it is. They don't beat around the bush. Some of the questions they ask you are classics.

One little girl once said, 'Did you have your accident messing around with trees?'

I said that I had. To which she replied, 'Well, you're not that great then are you?'

What could I say to that?

I had just been shot down in flames by a 6-year-old kid!

I spoke at one school and was warned the children there were on the verge of getting into trouble. I was a little apprehensive but told the staff I could be as harrowing as they wanted, or as mellow as they wanted. If they wanted me to scare some of the kids, I could do that. They told me to be mellow. By the end of the day, the children had formed an orderly queue for autographs and said, 'Thank you'. They were great.

The school was three miles away from the beach, yet most of these kids had never seen the sea. They were on a rough estate. The school was a lovely, brand new building as the old one had been burnt down. I had four 'sporting champions' T-shirts to give away at the school. To get one, a kid had to answer a question correctly about something I had discussed during the day, just to see whether they had been paying attention. I had been warned about one lad; however, he had been no trouble whatsoever and I could see he really wanted a T-shirt.

I had one T-shirt remaining. My last question was, 'What is my tennis chair made of?'

His hand went up straight away. 'Titanium!' he shouted out.

He was correct and he got himself a T-shirt.

I was amazed, as I had spoken about my chair two hours earlier. He had clearly been sat there just taking everything in. Then, he very politely came over and asked me if I would sign the shirt for him. Moments like that show you that you can affect people in a positive way.

Some schools are different, though. In one some kids jumped in my tennis chair and shot off in it. I ended up searching round the place for ages to try and get it back.

Carl Moffatt

For part of my degree I did some work on wheelchair sports and Mark helped me out a lot with that. That was a big part of me getting through my degree and I did an interview with him about the lack of recognition for disabled sportspeople. He was superb. He listed what he had done compared to Tim Henman; no competition, yet Henman is a household name.

FINAL FINAL WORDS

Apologies for preaching, but the value of respect has decreased in today's society in my opinion. For example, there is a sense of confinement when you're in hospital for a long time as I was after my accident. You can't get out and, if you try, there's someone there to stop you – just like at a prison. Back in those days, you did as you were told. I remember a couple of mornings I told the nursing staff I wasn't getting up. No chance! I would soon be got up, dressed and sent to the gym. You had no choice but to do as you were told.

Nowadays it seems to me that society is just one big free for all and all because of so-called human rights. *What a load of rubbish!*

This is where my dislike of do-gooders comes in. I get asked 'what do I term a do-gooder?'

For me a do-gooder is someone who has nothing better to do with their life except stand up for, and makes excuses for 'persistent offenders'.

It annoys me when I hear that people working in teaching, nursing and caring are getting verbally and physically abused. I wouldn't do their job in a million years. If I were helping or caring for someone and they gave me abuse, I would be livid.

Sometimes their arty smarty 'everyone is oppressed' attitude drives me nuts. Human rights are good in certain circumstances but there is too much of this caring for the criminal attitude. You read about a kid in a young offender's institute being taken on all expenses trip to Jamaica because it will boost his confidence. Bloody hell, I had to break my neck to boost mine.

Anyway, back in the good old days, you did as you were told and, at the end of the day, it was for your own good. I think it's sad for society that respect has gone. Respect for property, respect for older people and so on. I don't want to sound like a 90-year-old but, when I was younger, you didn't mouth off to grown ups. Now some kids will tell you to eff off. There are teachers who used to give me the cane or a clip round the ear and, if I see them today, I still call them 'sir' because I still respect them.

I put the death of respect down to do-gooders. You can't discipline anyone nowadays. If I did anything wrong at school and a teacher gave me a cuff round the ear and I told my parents about it, they'd give me a clip as well because I'd obviously been misbehaving in the first place. I grew up with respect. You can't earn it these days because there is no form of discipline.

Parking spaces for the disabled is one area where you sometimes see that lack of respect despite the fact that everyone is supposed to care for us poor wheelchair folk. I went to the supermarket recently and was going to park in the last remaining disabled space. A young lad got there first in his car and parked up. I asked him if he had a blue badge; he said he didn't, so I asked him to move, as I needed to park there.

He politely asked, 'Who the fuck are you?'

I told him I was a cripple who needed the parking spot. He told me ever so nicely to fuck off.

I caught up with him, and told him exactly what I thought of him, really lost my rag with the little shit. He was shocked. The irony of the situation was that as I was leaving the store, he ran after me and apologised.

ECCY'S CREED

If I can just help one person to think more positively, then that's an achievement.

If one person who is thinking of going the way of the despairing man in the bed opposite to me in the Spinal Unit, reads this book and it makes them go the other way, then it has been more than worth it. The ability to have a positive affect on someone's life is quite something.

One thing that irritates me is when someone who hasn't got a disability tells someone who has got a disability what they can, or can't, do. Do you want to know what it's like in my shoes? Then have an epidural in your back. It will be the worst hours of your life. Do you have to remember to shift your arse off your chair every five minutes to avoid pressure sores? Bet you don't!

With my tennis and rugby record you could argue I was one of the best all-round tetraplegic athletes, although a certain American would definitely come into the frame.

Rick Draney.

If you had a dream tournament of the best eight, true, tetraplegic tennis players ever then I believe the final would be between Draney and me and I think that he would win. (And before anyone says anything I said *true* tetras.)

I saw that man turn games round that he should not have been able to win. Tactically, he was better than anyone I've ever seen. He had a fantastic serve, the best forehand, a good backhand and was just a clever player who had great awareness. It took me about three years of hard work to beat him.

There are rugby players who were better than me, but who couldn't play tennis as well as me, such as Joe Soares. Whenever I played him in rugby he would always talk trash and when he won, he would always say, 'Get that shit out of here, you're in my house now.'

However, when I played him at tennis, I don't think he won a point – never mind a game.

Guess what I said to him at the end?

Also there are better tennis players than me that couldn't match me at wheelchair rugby. Brian Hanson springs to mind.

I have had a good ride and I've had a good laugh. Some people have the misconception that the quality of life of someone who has a spinal cord injury is reduced but attitudes are changing, I'm glad to say.

The positive, if you can take a positive out of me having my accident at the age of 16, was that I hadn't seen or done much at that point. I was in hospital with people who had accidents in later life. People who had experienced a hell of a lot and, all of a sudden, they had a spinal injury and were stuck in a wheelchair. It must have been harder for them in that respect. I hadn't experienced much at all when my life changed forever.

Now I have been in a wheelchair for over twenty years, longer than I was on my feet. It is a bizarre feeling, because I can still remember what it's like to walk and run, and kick a ball. I can remember those feelings. Whenever I have a dream I'm on my feet, and I often dream about rugby. I don't know whether that means that subconsciously I haven't accepted being in a wheelchair, but it's extremely annoying to wake up only to realise it was actually a dream.

I want to alter the general perception of what people in wheelchairs are like – and what they can, or can't, do.

I want to show that, just because I am in wheelchair, it doesn't limit my life. I've probably done more than most people my age.

I want people to see it's not all doom and gloom.

If someone is down, I don't want them reading this book and start crying their eyes out. I want someone to read it and realise that no matter your situation in life, no matter how bad it seems, there is always light at the end of the tunnel. There is something that you can do, something that you can achieve although it's going to take hard work. I have achieved a great deal, and it has been a lot of hard work, but so is anything worth having in life.

Writing this book has fired me up. What you have got to understand about me is that if I have something to say, I am not going to bite my lip! And that has pissed off a lot of people over the years.

Whatever opportunities come your way in life, if they are going to add value to you, you should take them. If it is something that is going to contribute positives to your life, then you have to take the opportunity.

I've had bad days and weeks where I think I've had enough. When you're having a hard time, you have to believe that you will be okay when you get through it.

I've always worked on the theory that, if you do get through the bad days, then the good days will taste even sweeter, and the sun will feel warmer. A lot of people are not as mentally strong as I am, and I'm not as mentally strong as a lot of other people; but whatever adversity life throws at you, rise to the challenge and meet it head on.

I always say that before my accident there were a million things that I could do. After my accident, there were 900,000 things I could do and a hundred thousand things I couldn't. Am I going to worry about the stuff I can't do – when there's so much that I can?

Even if I hadn't had my accident, would I have got through the million things anyway? I doubt it.

Even though, at times, everything seems dark and down, there are still things you can cling to and get on with. There are still things now I haven't done that I want to do. There is no point in worrying about the past, or things you can't control. You're only on this earth for 70 or 80 years, if you're lucky. Why waste that time on 'what ifs?' I'm too busy ploughing through the 900,000 things I can do to dwell on what might have been.

The one thing I wanted to do most both before and after my accident was to snorkel on the Great Barrier Reef, and I did it with Johnno in 2002. It was the best thing I have ever done. We had a two-hour cruise up the coast from Cairns past beautiful tropical rainforest. We then went to Agincourt Reef where there was a floating platoon with a chair, which you sat in, and they lowered you down. An amazing experience!

Sister Mary, the nun who saw me in hospital when I had my accident, used to say, 'Be happy today, be sad tomorrow.'

It's still one of the wisest things anyone has ever said to me.

When tomorrow comes, it's today and you have to be happy. Whenever I'm down I think of that saying. Tomorrow never comes.

It's like goal setting. When you achieve one goal, move on to the next one. That's relevant to sport and to life. If you want to achieve something, set yourself a realistic target. If you're not as confident or determined (or cocky) as me then you just set yourself a shorter target. Worry about tomorrow when it comes, but remember, tomorrow never comes – so why worry?

As far as future goals for myself, I would like a place somewhere warm to nip off to on a weekend. I suffer with the cold, probably old age kicking in.

Since packing in my sporting career, I feel I am still looking for that big something that I can focus on. I seem to be in limbo at the moment, although coaching does fire me up. This is understandable, as for the last 15 years it's been full on training, competing and setting goals.

I think it may be a little bit of 'after the Lord Mayor's show' feeling.

At the end of the day, you can't get better than being the best person on the planet at what you do. Things after that can seem a little small.

That's not to say there's not stuff I can be doing, I'm sure there is and I'm sure I will discover it.

When I look back from the initial time in hospital to where I am today, what a difference. At 16 I hated leaving the hospital and going home. Now I moan if I have to go back to the hospital for a check up.

After the accident, I made a decision never to give in. I made a choice. I thought if I took the wrong option and did give in, then it was a long time to be miserable – and it would make a lot of other people miserable too.

So I decided to do something with my life. My mum and dad did a fantastic job of raising my brothers and me. We're all happy and we've never been in trouble with the law, but if someone tells me I can't do something, I will usually go out of my way just to prove them wrong.

Sometimes I look at my brothers and my mates and feel I would swap all my sporting success to have the life they have. Maybe they sit there thinking they'd wish they'd travelled the world like me. The grass is always greener on the other side, I suppose.

Breaking your neck at sixteen is a devastating thing to have to deal with. I thought my world had ended and, if I am honest, I sometimes wished it had.

But if, when I lay in intensive care with weights attached to my head and paralysed, you had come in and said to me that I would go on to be World No 1, World Champion and Paralympics silver medallist, I would have laughed at you and told you where to go.

Now I would tell you to look at the CV.

Ian Moffatt

If you mention Mark Eccleston's name in Clock Face, the overwhelming response is one of respect. If you mean something to him, he has a heart of gold; if you don't, then forget it. As long as I have known him he has never suffered fools.

My dad used to say to me to motivate me, 'Look at Eccy', because he wanted me to be successful. Eccy and me have always been close; my family and his were close because we grew up together. The strength of his character is quite unique. I've never met a fella like him and the inner strength he possesses is quite incredible.

He is an absolute star and I could never say a bad word about him, which for me is very rare. I've had parents come crying to me saying how much he has inspired their kids. It's a sad thing that wheelchair sport has never been properly recognised. What he has put into wheelchair sport should have made him a household name.

He was the best tennis player in the world; he'll probably be the best tennis coach around, and if he flew a plane, he'd probably be best at that too!

If I can be successful and achieve my goals, then anyone can. I was just a kid thrust into a situation I didn't want to be in.

I made the decision I would do something with my life. I had a dream and went for it.

You don't have to be World No 1 to be successful. You can be the best in your class, or your school, or your work place.

If you set yourself a goal and you achieve it, then that's just as big an achievement as anything I ever did.

I am nothing special.

If I were, I would never have been World No 1. I would never have won a World Team Cup and I would never have won a Paralympic Silver Medal.

If I were anything special, you would not be reading this book and you might never have even heard of me.

Why?

Because, if I were special, then I would have nailed that somersault. In fact, if I were special, I wouldn't have tried it in the first place.

Chapter 21

The Record

RUGBY LEAGUE

1986   St Helens Crusaders Player of the year (runner-up)

TABLE TENNIS

1987   Silver medal. National Wheelchair Games
1988   Gold medal. National Wheelchair Games

WHEELCHAIR RUGBY

SOUTHPORT
1992   National Champions

SUNCOAST STORM (TAMPA 1994)
Silver medal. South Central Regional, Houston, USA
All star Team. South Central Regional, Houston, USA,
4th place National Championship, Boston USA

GREAT BRITAIN
1991   Selected for Great Britain tour to Dallas, USA
1992   Selected for Great Britain tour to Toronto, Canada
1993   Bronze medal. Tampa tournament (as captain)
1993   Bronze medal. Toronto tournament (as captain)
1993   Silver medal. International Games (as captain)

1994   Silver medal. International games (as captain)

1996   4th place. Paralympic Games, Atlanta (as captain)

WHEELCHAIR TENNIS (Quad division)

First British player ever to be World No 1 in singles from Feb 2003–Apr 2004

First British player ever to be world No 1 in doubles 1999

SINGLES
National Champion: 1995, 1996, 1997, 1998, 2000, 2001, 2002
British Open: Winner 1995
US Indoor, Milwaukee: Winner 1998
Australian Open Winner: 2001 ,2002
Sydney Open: Winner 2001, 2002
Florida Open: Winner 2002
Belgium Open: Winner 2002
Japan Open: Winner 1998, 2000
Dutch Open: Winner 2000
Czech indoor: Winner 2002
Nottingham Indoor: Winner 2003

DOUBLES
US Outdoor Championship, Atlanta: Winner 1997
Dutch Open: Winner 1998, 2000, 2004
British Open: Winner 1998
Japan Open: Winner 2000, 2001
Sydney International: Winner 2001
Belgium Open: Winner 2001
Swiss Open: Winner 2001, 2004
Lakeshore Challenge, Alabama: Winner 2002
Florida Open: Winner 2003
Australian Open: Winner 2004
Athens Paralympics 2004: Silver Medal

WORLD TEAM CUP (Davis Cup of Wheelchair Tennis)

1998   Barcelona, Spain: Runner up

2001   Sion, Switzerland: Winner

2002   Tremosine, Italy: Winner

2003   Sopot, Poland: Runner up

INTERNATIONAL WHEELCHAIR TENNIS RECORD

	Played	Won	Lost
SINGLES	163	107	56
DOUBLES	104	67	37

AWARDS

2002   North West Disabled Athlete of the Year
          LTA Disabled Player of the Year

2001   Dan Maskell Player's Player of the Year 1999, 2001
          NWTA Men's Player of the Year 2002
          2 BWSF Awards

AV IT!!!!

Editor: Reuben Cohen

The publisher wishes to thank Sonia Land
of Sheilland Associates for her help

A DVD of
Pushing the Limits
is available from
Psychology News Ltd
9a Artillery Passage, London E1 7LN
Price £12.99